A to Z
Mini-Guide to Women's Health

A to Z
Mini-Guide to Women's Health

Karen Stone

Copyright 2017 Karen Stone
Registered at Copyright house

All rights reserved.

Typesetting and kindle formatting by Word-2-kindle

ISBN: 978-1-5272-0872-8

First edition Ebook January 2017
First edition Paperback May 2017

Cover by Sean@perception-marketing.co.uk

DISCLAIMER

This book is not intended as a substitute for the medical advice of physicians. The reader should regularly consult a physician in matters relating to her health, and particularly with respect to any symptoms that may require diagnosis or medical attention.

CONTENTS

PREFACE 9
A to Z mini-guide 15

AIR-BRUSHED 17
ALCOHOL 21
ALTERNATIVES 24
ANTI OXIDANTS 28
BOWELS 33
BRAIN 40
BREASTS 47
CHEMICALS 54
CHI 60
CHOCOLATE 62
CHLAMYDIA 64
COCONUT MILK AND OIL 70
CONTRACEPTIVES 72
DEBT 75
DETOX DAY 78
DIARY 82
DRUGS 84
ESSENTIAL OILS 91
EXERCISE 101
FASTING 105
FERTILITY 108
FISH 111

FOOD	113
GARLIC	118
GENETICALLY ENGINEERED	120
GOALS	122
GRATITUDE	126
GREEN TEA	129
HERBS	130
HORMONES	140
IRON	149
JUICING	150
KINDNESS	155
LOVE	156
MEDITATION AND MINDFULNESS	159
MEN	163
MENOPAUSE	165
MINERALS	175
NUTS	178
OMEGAS	179
OSTEOPOROSIS	181
OVARIES	186
PRODUCTS	189
QIGONG	193
RECIPES	194
RELATIONSHIPS	206
SEX	209
SKIN	212
SLEEP	219
SUGAR	221
THOUGHTS	227
TOXIC	229
URINARY	233
US	235
UTERUS	237

VAGINA	241
VEGETABLES	247
VITAMINS	255
WATER	257
WORDS OF WISDOM	261
XYLITOL	269
YOGA	271
ZINC	280
CONTENTS	283
BIBLIOGRAPHY AND RECOMMENDED READING	287
ACKNOWLEDGEMENTS	289

PREFACE

I've written this book as I have always been passionate and fascinated with the human body, mind and spirit. Our bodies and minds have an innate, miraculous capacity to self heal given the right conditions and attitude. We all need to take responsibility to care for ourselves.

I'm fifty two now and am still curious, reading and studying. I wasn't academic at school and I don't have a degree but have always read voraciously. I went to technical college full time when I was eighteen, to train as a beauty and massage therapist. Whilst there, I studied anatomy and physiology to a high level, which has been helpful in my other role as a yoga teacher. We also studied some cosmetic chemistry. I have an ITEC qualification in Aromatherapy and studied nutrition myself for ten years.

I worked as a therapist for thirty years and it was invaluable in the way it taught Service. To listen closely to women, to empathise and to either relax them or to lift their self esteem in whatever small way we could, is a skill in itself.

In my mid thirties a friend of my mother's, who I shall always be grateful to, suggested that I train as a yoga teacher. My mum has always practised yoga and still does every day. It was a natural progression as I had been practising yoga from the age of sixteen, along with martial art classes. I started to read yogic philosophy in my early twenties and had experienced different styles and teachers by the time I went to train. My initial course was a month long Sivanander teacher training course and from that point I attended as many day, weekend, week courses and teacher training sessions as I could. I went to Iyengar, Integral, Ashtanga, dynamic Vinyasa flow yoga classes over the next ten years appreciating and admiring them all.

These days I enjoy a still, restorative Yin practise and am practising Qigong. Everything is linked up when you yoke physical movement with breath awareness. Different practises correlate and have similarities to take you towards a still, peaceful mind and state.

I've been teaching yoga for the last sixteen years which is fulfilling, but can be challenging, as to be self employed you need to be resilient. You must stay motivated and positive as a sole trader and to adapt and adjust. You're responsible for not only planning the class and executing it clearly, whilst attempting to make it enjoyable, but also for keeping up to date with accounts, balancing books, marketing and advertising. Traversing the web and I.T has been a huge challenge for me. Assessing a large group of people with assorted ages, physical injuries or problems and health issues is part of the job. We aspire to presenting them with a class that they feel is accessible, yet challenging enough and safe.

After years of teaching, boredom can set in, so we need to inspire and refresh ourselves. Life is like this. To carry on you need to become a little thick skinned, to try not to take things personally and to put what you consider to be a temporary failure behind you.

PREFACE

On my journey in my own body and mind I've had to deal with health problems, chronic fatigue syndrome (M.E), debt, miscarriage, long distance relationships and divorce. Most of us will traverse life with some setbacks and disappointments, but life is beautiful, profound and a huge learning curve. Life is a giant school. "Failure" is another chance to get up, dust yourself off, re-focus and just keep on keeping on.

The menopause has been a gargantuan challenge. I have currently decided not to take HRT but to continue to invest in supplements and alternatives. Be kind to women who appear to be scowling, have lost their way in more ways than one and are rubbing their midriffs in an attempt to find the waist they once had, which has disappeared along with their sense of humour, energy and concentration.

Be yourself. You'll find that most people will like you, but some just won't. Recognise that none of us are perfect, we're human. I have always struggled from a very young age with jealously and being overly sensitive to criticism. We get to know ourselves as we mature and can gently observe our egos.

Our physical and mental health may oscillate through our lives. A great many women suffer with mental health issues but the taboo is lessening. We need to give ourselves time to heal, to accept where we are and to make the best of ourselves and what we have.

We're not just bags of skin around a bony frame, filled in with water and sparking electrical impulses. Running through us is an intelligence that is a light we need to lovingly observe and connect with on a regular basis. Call that light whatever you like, a flame, soul or spirit, it integrates with the rest of us. It's well known that the physical body is linked to mind and spirit and that they interconnect and subtly influence each other. Yogic philosophy regards the individual as connected and interdependent with everyone. Each person though, has "layers" around them, akin to an onion. Firstly, the material body of joints, muscle and bone, the mental body with thoughts leading to emotions, the importance and profundity of breath and a bliss "layer", a state beyond duality.

Finally, I wrote this book in the hope that it will guide and inspire teenagers and women in their early twenties to care for themselves on all levels. Some of the chapters are specifically for teenagers and a few other chapters just for women in their late forties. The sections pertaining to diet, nutrition, food, exercise, mindfulness within movement and spiritualism are for all women of all ages. I would like this mini guide to be passed between mother and daughter, then discussed with your cousin or aunty, so that it is shared knowledge.

Life should be fun and it is about making mistakes and making decisions. Make plans through your life and enjoy them whether they bear fruit or not. Recognise when something's not working for you or supporting or fulfilling you. Forgive people whenever you can, as quickly as you can, because hurt is a bitter pill that ultimately poisons only you. Stay cheerful and grateful. Accept with good grace whatever comes your way, but develop courage and belief in yourself so that you can walk another path if you need to. Speak up when you need to.

The women in your life; family, friends and colleagues can be a support network and enrich and enliven your life. Invest time and love into these relationships, but take

PREFACE

the time to chat to strangers sometimes too. Whatever you put in eventually comes back to you.

A TO Z MINI-GUIDE

The A to Z mini-guide for women's health blends physical, mental, emotional and spiritual knowledge and offers advice to inspire you to make decisions through all the stages of your life so that you can live optimally. Decisions you make as a teenager, in your twenties and later as you move through life into menopause and after, will enhance your experience. It will make transitions smoother, promoting your longevity and contentment. As a reference book it's easy to read, highly informative and contains some of the latest research. As you read through it the words that are in CAPITALS are chapter headings so that you can cross reference and find out more about that subject and research it further.

It is relevant for women of all ages and is simple to apply in everyday life. I have also written this guide to educate and inspire young women between the ages of fourteen and twenty one who are contemplating a career as a nurse, therapist, physiotherapist, nutritionist, sports trainer, yoga, Pilates teacher or beautician.

We are not just physical beings. Holistic health and well being needs to be approached from all angles. This book will be an inspiration to move through challenges and towards being the best that you can be with optimal health.

A TO Z MINI-GUIDE

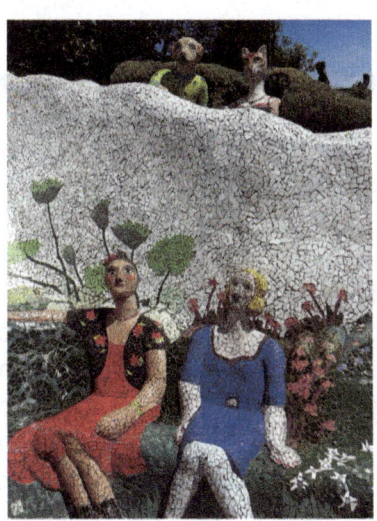

AIR-BRUSHED

As far as physical appearance goes, I have a fairly large, crooked nose with horse sized nostrils, a wide, square, almost manly jaw and very thin, narrow lips. When someone takes a photo of me you can see that, if it's a wide smile, one of my front teeth is a little crooked and my teeth slightly yellow. I used to be a size ten, but am now a size fourteen. I am tall though, and have been told I'm handsome and striking with curvy buttocks, long legs and deep green eyes, which are my redeeming feature.

Most of us are a little vain but appearance isn't everything. We are self deprecating and dislike parts of ourselves, our faces and bodies, scrutinizing them every now and again. We can make the most of our good points. Our smiles, if they are genuine, can light up our faces. We are beautiful in our uniqueness and it's fun to play with our image. Confidence is beautiful.

Advertising and media have set women up to compare themselves with images which are prolific, unreal and for most of us, unobtainable and unrealistic. There is software available to "air-brush" photos and images. They remove "imperfections" and erase fine, facial lines or cellulite on thighs. We forget this when a billboard advertising lingerie comes into view. Advertising is always telling us that we are lacking in some way that we would be so much happier, popular and loved if we bought a certain product. It's manipulation that we all buy into. We're hardwired from an early age.

From as young as six, girls are becoming aware of weight, image and clothes. We do need to maintain awareness of obesity as it is detrimental to health, becoming obese does not happen overnight. Anorexia and bulimia are linked to mental health and an unreal image. We need patience and compassion to help young women overcome them.

The attitude to Body Mass Index (BMI) and the amount of fat you carry may be changing. Can you be a size sixteen, have healthy levels of cholesterol, exercise every day and still be considered unhealthy? Very overweight and very underweight people will probably have a lower life expectancy. Weight around your belly and organs is a marker for ill health so if you're an "apple" shape and not a "pear" take steps to lose some of this fat.

The three types of body are; ectomorph, mesomorph and endomorph and how you look may be partly genetic. Find your ideal weight so that you can move easily and freely, exercise regularly and eat and drink with moderation. Professionals can check your heart rate, blood pressure and cholesterol levels regularly, so use these as markers for health.

AIR-BRUSHED

I buy the fashion magazine Marie Claire most months. This may sound contrary but I enjoy making clothes, wearing eye shadow and I've had purple hair. Every day I apply concealer under my eyes and peach blusher on my cheeks as I feel I look brighter and a little better. I remind myself that the world of fashion and beauty is surreal as I flick through the magazine. I'm glad to see a "plus" size female journalist with her own page for recommending clothes. This beautiful woman is advocating figure hugging prints. I feel it's a step in the right direction to start to move away from using size zero models. I wonder what it must be like to eat a spoonful of yogurt and a lettuce leaf for dinner all month. I read most of Marie Claire but in particular find the articles about women in different cultures and situations informative. At times they are harrowing and at times, uplifting. Become aware of what is going on in the world and issues that involve the well being of women globally. Step outside of your own little world and get informed. Whether you just sign a petition every now and again or get involved with charities, you're broadening your knowledge about women and their various plights. Issues like Female Genital Mutilation are no longer being airbrushed or ignored as groups are campaigning against abuse.

As women, we can enjoy enhancing ourselves. It's up to us how far we take that. I recently read that women in their late twenties are having Botox and cosmetic fillers. Research all the options if you are thinking about it and go online to inform yourself of pitfalls and incidences when surgery went very wrong. Enhancement is a personal decision and can boost self esteem, just be aware that you are "air-brushing" yourself. Try not to compare yourself too much with other women as it could make you either vain or despondent. Make the best of yourself.

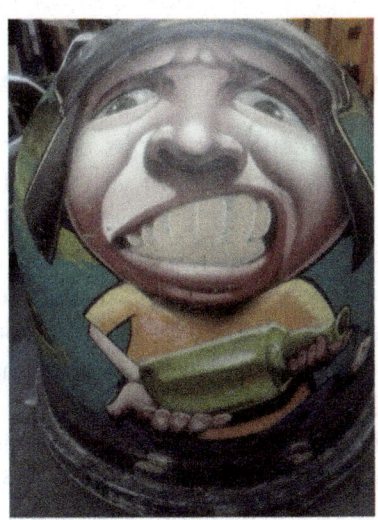

ALCOHOL

Alcohol can be celebratory and has ancient, tribal connections. Whether it's been made from potatoes or sloe berries it can cheer us. It can lift gatherings and make our taste buds sing.

As with everything, moderation is the key. There is a dark side to alcohol. If you use it regularly in excess just to switch off from a stressful job and drink to oblivion so that you can finally sleep, you need other options.

Happy hours and binge drinking have resulted in higher than ever visits to Accident and Emergency in city centres resulting in long queues and three to four hours of painful, wasted, waiting around for those people in need of medical aid. Most of us like a drink or two, but if you have a habit of a Gin and tonic or three or a bottle of wine every night, take a break. Your liver needs to work hard to process everything, so have one or two "dry" days a week.

Alcohol is a central nervous system depressant, so you could feel more tired if you overdo it. If you're going through MENOPAUSE a few cocktails won't really help if you have hot flushes, as alcohol can aggravate them. Excessive alcohol affects your bone density which ultimately leads to OSTEOPOROSIS. If you drink most evenings, you increase your risk of dealing with seven different types of cancer.

The incidence of women in their forties becoming drunk and disorderly in the streets has been rising. Eat something before you head out and give yourself a limit, particularly if you're feeling emotionally low, as they're the times we find solace in alcohol.

Some of us will have gone through our late teens and twenties drunk on large bottles of cider or home mixed cocktails. It is a rite of passage for a lot of people. Experimenting with a lack of regard for the risks is part of growing up. If you're in your late teens or early twenties, go to parties with friends and always keep an eye on each other. Our twenties can be fun and alcohol invariably plays a part in it, just have days when you don't indulge at all. Drink a large mug of water before you go to bed after a night out to avoid dehydration.

Drinking alcohol and taking DRUGS can be escapism from emotional pain or situations we can't face or deal with. Don't succumb to peer-pressure if you are not comfortable with getting so drunk you pass out. If you get into a car and you know the driver has had a few, you're gambling with your life. You might think it won't happen to you but it could, and it's your family and friends who would grieve. DRUGS will also take you over an acceptable limit for driving, so if you value the freedom that your licence gives you, think twice.

ALCOHOL

Marijuana and alcohol could still be in your system when you get in your car the next morning.

Medical studies and experts may reach a point where they conclude that blood sugar levels are linked to alcoholism, which is a disease in which you find it almost impossible to get through a day without booze.

The good news is that Resveratrol, an ANTIOXIDANT found in grapes, red wine and berries has anti aging properties. A recent study showed that even with a diet of fatty food, the resveratrol increased the effectiveness of the immune system by boosting levels of T cells, an integral part of immune function. It also stimulated the growth of new mitochondria which are the "engines" in our cells, creating energy from the food we eat. Mitochondria are damaged by free radicals as we age, so by drinking a few small glasses of red wine a week, we can repair our bodies at a cellular level!

White wine tends to have more additives and Sulphites which can cause headaches in some people, so switch to red for the benefits of resveratrol. If you're watching weight and counting calories, have a glass of champagne or a small vodka and cranberry juice as a weekly treat.

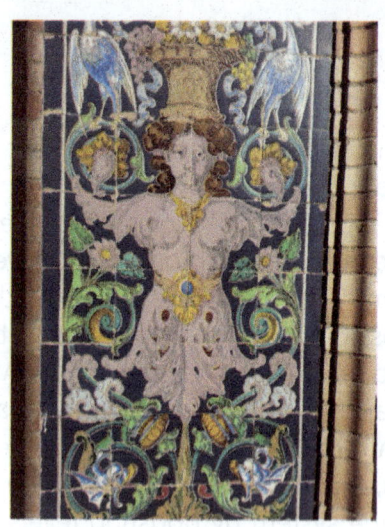

ALTERNATIVES

There may be times in our lives when we will be prescribed pharmaceutical drugs and pain killers. More and more doctors and general practitioners are recommending, after consideration, other options. Here are a few of them.

Acupuncture is a few thousand years old and originates from Asia. Due to the toxicity and addictive nature of some pharmaceutical DRUGS, this is an alternative option which for many people, suffering with a wide range of illnesses and painful conditions, have found relief as endorphins are released during treatment. Get a recommendation from someone who's been to one. When you go for a consultation and treatment, fine needles will be inserted into specific acupuncture points. Read the chapters on CHI and QIGONG for more background information about Eastern practises. Acupuncture promotes self healing by the body and your systems. The needles are placed into the surface of the SKIN and work by releasing blockages of energy in meridians or energy channels. The needles stay in for between five and thirty minutes and are normally not painful. The acupuncturist will inform you of how many treatments they feel you need. This is no longer just ancient philosophy, as scientists are researching it. If you live in Britain contact the British Acupuncture Council.

We become uneven (mentally and physically) through our lives because of repetitive movements or unhealthy habits. Chronic pain from injuries can cause referred pain as the body tries to re-stabilise. An Alexander technique teacher will assess you and ask you to participate in a one to one lesson, where you'll learn ease in movement, with minimal tension or unnecessary force. The teacher will approach your lesson with a holistic view and knowledge that mind and body are linked together for optimal health and comfort. The aim, with the client's ongoing awareness, is to improve coordination, balance and stability. The Alexander technique can alleviate muscular stiffness and tension in your back, improve vocal and breathing capabilities, re-educate your mind and body to heighten postural ease in every day movements and reduce stress.

There are many different kinds of massage available. Swedish massage improves blood circulation and muscular aches and pains and is the root of many other massage techniques. It should be soothing and relaxing. Serotonin and dopamine are neurotransmitters in the BRAIN, massage helps to elevate them bringing contentment. Massage also lowers levels of the hormone arginine vasopressin which helps to regulate blood pressure. It can be an aid in decreasing levels of the stress HORMONE cortisol which increases belly fat. Putting weight on around your midriff can be an indicator of heart disease.

Lymphatic drainage massage utilises a technique which is very light. This is effective where there is an issue with fluid retention and lymphoedema, or if you have had certain lymph nodes removed. It is a specialised draining technique and is said to alleviate pain in people with fibromyalgia. It benefits the lymphatic system which carries the lymph fluid containing our white blood cells around the body. Our lypmphatic system is part of our immune response.

Aromatherapy uses ESSENTIAL OILS blended after a consultation to ascertain your mental, emotional and physical state. A form of sweeping massage is then used with the oils blended specifically for you.

Deep tissue massage uses techniques with more intense pressure applied to muscles, fascia and tendons. If there has been the formation of scar tissue this type of massage helps to break it up, so loosening and freeing that specific area.

Sports massage therapists will not give you a soothing, relaxing treatment as their aim is to re-establish optimal motion and movement in impaired joints and muscles. They can give you a program to practise every day to heal injuries and for rehabilitation.

Myofascial release massage has its main focus on the joints and fascia, which is the fibrous tissue that surrounds everything in the body. Myofascial treatment concentrates more on the soft tissue in the body, improving range of movement in joints, which may be helpful for people with fibromyalgia.

Tui na is an Asian form of fairly vigorous deep tissue massage linked to CHI and the removal of blockages

ALTERNATIVES

along meridian channels. When stagnant chi or energy doesn't flow, pain and disease can set in. Some of the techniques used in Tui na are similar to western massage and alleviate muscular pain, but acupressure points are also used to rebalance mental and physical conditions. It is a holistic approach. Chronic stress leads to disease and massage lowers the effects of stress. Acupuncture and the use of HERBS may also be used in Tui na.

Thai massage comprises of rocking, stretching and pressing movements. The therapist performs this treatment on the floor, enabling them to manipulate the client into various positions whilst they apply pressure with their hands, elbows or feet. This is excellent for muscular pain and stress. The client remains fully clothed.

I have Reflexology regularly and find it deeply relaxing and calming and beneficial for imbalances on many levels. It involves lying down whilst a therapist uses finger and thumb techniques across your feet. The points on your feet correlate to organs and systems as well as your spine. It has been particularly good for sinusitis.

ANTI OXIDANTS

Free radicals are molecules that have an unstable electron which can damage DNA and cells in your body. They are partly produced as a result of us needing lots of oxygen. If you regularly run or do a lot of aerobic exercise you may need to increase anti oxidants. The vitamins A, C and E are anti oxidants as they counteract the damage, but there are many other plants and sources which act in this way.

VITAMIN A is known as retinol or carotene and is required to absorb calcium for healthy bones and teeth. It is linked to night vision, aiding the immune system and to keeping the genito-urinary tract, the throat, nose lining, digestive and respiratory lining healthy. Beta carotene comes in the form of eggs and dairy products which are absorbed in the small intestine and converted into Vitamin A. If you don't eat cheddar cheese, butter, cream, eggs or milk because you are vegan, you may need to supplement.

VITAMIN C comes in a few different forms, one of which is ascorbate. Ascorbic is another. A mix of magnesium ascorbate, calcium ascorbate and ascorbyl palmitate is known to be easily assimilated. It maintains the capillary walls in blood vessels, heals SKIN when damaged or burnt, as it is essential in the formation of collagen (the connective part of flesh), and keeps gums

ANTI OXIDANTS

healthy. Many people take Vitamin C as a supplement and it's needed for the body to absorb vitamin A, IRON and folic acid. As an additive in food in Europe it's labelled as E300. Best food sources are raw red and green peppers, kiwis, onions, citrus fruit, prunes, Brussels sprouts, leafy green vegetables and blackcurrants. Unless they're stored in a dark fridge they will lose their vitamin C content in a day or two.

Steam your vegetables to ensure the optimal amount of vitamin C and use fresh or frozen instead of canned. If you have high levels of stress you will have more of the HORMONE cortisol in your system. This can lead to more fat around your belly which is a warning sign for health. Take 1000mg of vitamin C a day with your multi VITAMIN and MINERAL supplement to offset cortisol.

Vitamin E is known as a-tocopherol and also strengthens the walls of blood capilliaries, and may protect against heart disease and cancer. The best form to take as a supplement is natural source d-alpha tocopheryl succinate. The best food sources are almonds and cashew nuts, sweet potatoes, avocados and brown rice. If you're struggling with MENOPAUSE an extra vitamin E supplement will help.

Selenium and ZINC are also powerful antioxidants so read the chapter on MINERALS to find out how to get them into your diet.

Glutathione is produced in our bodies through our lives. It is made up of three amino acids, glutamine, cysteine and glycine, which are essential proteins. Glutathione contains sulphur which helps to battle free radicals and aids in the removal of heavy metals in the body. (If you're having mercury fillings removed, go to a specialist dentist). Thousands of nutritional studies have been carried out and shown glutathione to be a powerful detoxifier, anti-oxidant and free radical scavenger. Free radicals are randomly breaking down our cells daily from a combination of poor diet, lack of EXERCISE or too much exercise, and stress.

Due to pollution, CHEMICALS and TOXINS, our systems become challenged and unable to use or produce glutathione, so levels in our bodies become depleted. This is thought to contribute to disease and illness. If you suffer with diabetes, chronic fatigue syndrome, cancer, Alzheimer's and autoimmune disease you could consider taking steps to increase levels of glutathione. By taking a multi VITAMIN and MINERAL containing the B complex and selenium in particular, you boost your body into producing glutathione. Glutathione re-uses the antioxidants VITAMIN C and E and helps to reduce inflammation, which is a marker in the body for chronic disease.

To increase your levels of glutathione ensure you EXERCISE at least a few times a week for twenty five minutes. Include these VEGATABLES in your diet; watercress, cabbage, broccoli, kale, GARLIC and onions. If you're taking supplements, alpha lipoic acid and n-acetyle-cysteine will boost glutathione and your general health.

There are a number of powerful antioxidants that can be taken as supplements as we age or if the immune system is compromised. I recently read articles regarding ashwangara, an Ayurvedic Indian plant that has been shown in tests to enhance the nerve impulses and connections in the BRAIN so could be useful in treating Alzheimer's. It also stabilizes HORMONES and may be useful during MENOPAUSE.

ANTI OXIDANTS

Curcumin, the active ingredient in Turmeric may also be effective for keeping BREAST tissue healthy, lowering inflammation in the joints and aiding the immune system in the brain. Curcumin will help to reduce bacteria in the BRAIN.

Coenzyme Q10 or Ubiquinone is sometimes included in a potent supplement or can be taken separately and is important for energy production as well as an antioxidant and for heart abnormalities. It may be helpful if you have Chronic Fatigue Syndrome or M.E.

Astaxanthin is an incredible red coloured anti-oxidant found in marine plants and animals. To get this nutrient in your weekly diet, eat krill, shrimps, trout, crab and wild pacific sockeye salmon. When you take it as a supplement it generally comes from microalgae. It can aid the immune system, lower the risk of cataracts in eyes, stabilise the heart and improve the texture of your SKIN.

Bioflavanoids in supplements increase the effectiveness and potency of other antioxidants. Another interesting product to take in regard to assisting the immune function is colloidal silver, which is supposed to be highly effective against bacteria, viruses and fungal infections. Certain strains of bacteria have become resistant to antibiotics, rendering them useless. Colloidal silver can be used on the skin, topically for cuts and infections and is used in hospitals. Take a teaspoon orally a few times a week if you have a chronic infection. This is a powerful alternative to antibiotics and should be used as a preventative too. It can be taken with antibiotics if you have to take a course. Always take acidophilus after antibiotics.

If your body is constantly fighting fungus, viruses and bacterial infection, the immune system won't be as effective at scavenging and destroying other abnormalities in your cells, which is what it does very well when you're in optimal health. Take a quality multi vitamin and mineral supplement every day. You can be tested to see if you are deficient in individual nutrients. Check the label for the most effective ingredients. Chelated MINERALS are highly recommended as some other forms are not easily absorbed.

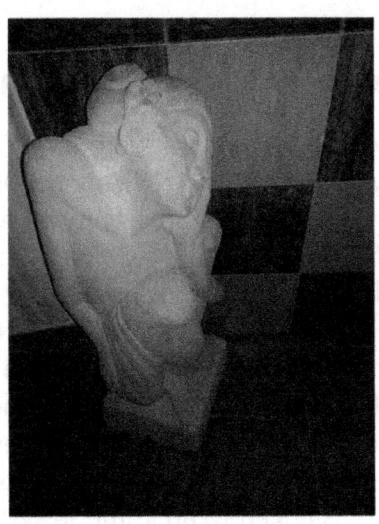

BOWELS

Eat plenty of fresh vegetables, some fruit, milled flax seed and a few nuts every day to ensure the health of your bowel. The smooth running and elimination of waste and toxins is essential for optimal health. Take a look at the contents of your bowel every now and again. Size, shape and colour of the stools are indicators of normality and health. Your stools should be smooth and soft, like a small sausage and be medium to light brown in colour. If they have excess mucous or blood in them, or are black or yellow and very narrow, consult your GP.

Gripping pain and discomfort can be signs that you have irritable bowel syndrome (IBS). This can start in your twenties and may be linked to stress or an inefficient immune system. Studies have shown that women who suffer with IBS had low levels of VITAMIN B6. Take a multi B complex supplement daily.

Diverticulitis is a condition where small pockets in the intestines become inflamed and infected because waste from food becomes trapped. Try to monitor your stress levels with a QIGONG, YOGA or MEDITATION class or relaxation techniques, as anxiety may be linked to the worsening of symptoms.

Colitis relates to problems and disease in the bowel. Crohn's disease causes inflammation in the digestive system. You're more likely to be diagnosed if you smoke and are a white European. Crohn's can be genetic, so passed through families. Additional causes and factors are a past severe infection and compromised micro biome. Crohn's is linked to an immune system response and reaction in the digestive tract.

The other condition where the bowel is inflamed is ulcerative colitis. The symptoms of Crohn's are; sore, red eyes, low appetite, weight loss, feeling run down and exhausted, abdominal pain, diarrhoea, joint pain and anaemia. If there is blood or pus in the diarrhoea inform your doctor. If you have been diagnosed you may be offered steroids and anti-inflammatory drugs or antibiotics.

Keep a FOOD DIARY, so that you record what you eat and drink every day, to see if symptoms link up to certain foods. Some foods and some beverages will exacerbate Crohn's. Dairy, wheat, red meat, spices, fried food, cabbage, broccoli, lentils, beans and chocolate, coffee and tea could cause a problem. Raw fruit and vegetables may also be problematic. Avoid too much ALCOHOL. Find alternative painkillers if you take them, as you also need to avoid ibuprofen and aspirin.

ESSENTIAL OILS can be helpful if bloated and constipated. Rub five drops of peppermint oil and five of ginger in a base oil of 20ml on your abdominal area, moving your hands from the left hip bone to the right hip bone, up to the right side of the rib cage, and across to the left side then back down to the left hip as firmly as you can following the bowel.

Occasional diarrhoea or constipation is normal if you're travelling abroad or dehydrated. Drink pure water during the day before meals, to ensure you avoid dehydration and have one or two bowel movements every day. Chew your food slowly and take time to stop and enjoy eating.

Antidepressants, antacids, IRON supplements and blood pressure medication contribute to constipation. Antibiotics, hormonal CONTRACEPTIVES and excessive SUGAR can disrupt your bowel or gut. We might occasionally need antibiotics if we have a severe bacterial infection. ESSENTIAL OILS of thyme, tea tree, clove and eucalyptus are also excellent at combating bacterial infections.

Antibiotics adversely affect our gut by destroying healthy 'flora' and good, beneficial bacteria in the bowel. Take a probiotic after a course of antibiotics and during the year, to top up the good bacteria which can be depleted from stress, medication and poor diet. Invest in a product that contains Lactobacillus acidophilus and L casei rhamnosus strains. When you buy a probiotic product look for these bacterial strains too ; bifidobacterium bifidum, Saccharomyces boulardii and Lactobacillus bulgaricus. We inadvertently ingest antibiotics in poultry and meat which may contribute to weight gain. Get creative with VEGETABLES, HERBS and cheese so you cut down on or eliminate red meat from your diet.

Ractopamine is a beta-agonist drug used to promote growth in animals which end up in your supermarket and on your plate. Beta-agonists are found in asthma medications and weight gain can be a factor if you take them. You can still enjoy meat a couple of times a week if you source it ethically. Ibuprofen and anti-inflammatory drugs can also destabilise the gut, causing bloating and discomfort.

An unhealthy gut can become 'leaky' or hyper permeable which leads to food particles getting into the bloodstream, and leading to food intolerances as your body tries to develop antibodies to sort this out. Those of you who have eczema or SKIN issues have different gut bacteria so look at food intolerances as an initial plan to control flare-ups. The fungus candida albicans can cause health problems if it is allowed to become prolific in the digestive system.

CAFOS are confined animal feeding operations where animals are injected with growth hormones which may have an oestrogenic effect and may increase your chance of dealing with breast cancer. Animals may be kept in unacceptable pens which are cramped and filthy and which increase the chances of infection. They are inhumane. Limit the amount of poultry and red meat you eat during the week.

Eat sauerkraut, tempeh and fermented foods every week and drink kumbuchu tea and apple cider vinegar to replenish and stabilise your bowel. The 'good' bacteria in your bowels, known as the micro biome, are linked to optimal physical and mental health and behaviour. Research is indicating that autism and depression may be connected to unstable, unbalanced micro biomes (the gut or bowel population of good bacteria).

Mothers who give birth naturally may have an advantage over those who opt for caesareans. As we pass through the birth canal and VAGINA we pick up our mother's vaginal microbes and this may be beneficial to our overall health later in life.

The gut is now regarded as the second brain as it houses the enteric nervous system (ENS). Our bowels contain the second largest number of neurocells in the body after the BRAIN. The ENS controls the activity of around thirty neurotransmitters. Dopamine and serotonin are neurotransmitters which elevate contentment, so are connected to a positive mood. Most of our serotonin is produced in the gut or bowel in the ENS. Bacterial waste products are also beneficial for the brain as they produce the neurotransmitter y-aminobutyric acid (GABA). Gaba and acetylcholine lower blood pressure and heart rate so that you can rest in a relaxed state.

The vagus nerve connects the BRAIN to the digestive area and is the longest nerve in the body. The vagus nerve starts in the brain from two main branches at the cerebellum, as cranial nerve ten. It moves down the neck, through the spleen, pancreas, liver, heart and lungs. Messages from your organs and 'gut' are sent up to the brain. Afferent nerve signals are sent from a nerve receptor into the brain. Efferent signals are sent from the brain to the body's systems. The vagus nerve connects into the 'gut' and micro biome, playing a role in stable mental health and the degree of inflammation in the body. Inflammation is detrimental to optimal health and is a marker for conditions such as endometriosis and the auto immune conditions of lupus, rheumatoid arthritis and bowel disease.

The vagus nerve works through the parasympathetic nervous system which initiates rest and relaxation, as opposed to the sympathetic nervous system of 'flight or fight', which releases a flood of adrenalin which may not be needed or disposed off. Constant stress can leave us feeling depleted due to us being unable to turn off this switch.

You can improve the tone and effectiveness of the vagus nerve by gradually improving your breathing techniques which are an essential part of YOGA practise, but can be used as part of a daily MINDFULNESS relaxation.

Vagal tone is measured by assessing the heart rate with your breathing rate. The bigger the difference between your inhalation and exhalation the higher your vagal tone is. If you regularly practise gentle but smooth, full inhalations followed by extended exhalations you will deal with stress more effectively. It sounds very simple and it is. Build up to this gradually without force or strain, after you've practised YOGA for a few months.

If you attend a YOGA class you'll learn pranayama, powerful breathing techniques which you can combine with affirmations, which are positive sentences you can repeat in your mind to enhance the connection between breathing deeply and feeling relaxed and calm. Try QIGONG or tai chi as forms of moving meditations.

This practise is essential if you suffer from ME, chronic fatigue syndrome, depression, heart conditions and diabetes, anxiety and adrenal burn out, but it will benefit anyone who wishes to stay calm and centred under pressure. Stress leads to ill health so take time to deeply relax.

Physical touch and stable, loving emotional connections with partners, friends and family will benefit the parasympathetic nervous system and the vagus nerve,

BOWELS

which is a link to the bowel and an important aspect of good health.

BRAIN

We take our good health for granted, but around our mid twenties we start to age, and our faculties in our fifties may not be as sharp as they were in our twenties. Our brains are made up mostly of fat and feed on sugar and oxygen. Oxidation is the unavoidable process of decay. It's akin to the rusting and rotting that you see in everyday life all around you and it's happening in our brains and bodies. The brain starts to show degeneration around our mid twenties and by our mid fifties, we can be forgetful and grumpy

Certain nutrients and food affect our mood. Protein will make us more alert than carbohydrates, so consider having eggs for breakfast and porridge after work or an hour before bed. We can raise the levels of the three neurotransmitters, serotonin, dopamine and norepinephrine (which are human chemicals in the brain), to feel more content and positive.

Serotonin lowers nervous anxiety and relaxes us and we can increase it by eating certain carbohydrates in small amounts. We need most of our carbohydrates from VEGETABLES. Avoid white rice, pasta, potatoes and too much bread. The amino acid tryptophan and vitamin B6 also contribute to raising serotonin levels so eat more chicken, (free range and ethically sourced), seeds and NUTS.

BRAIN

Dopamine and norepinephrine energise the brain to boost motivation, so having protein before work or when you have to focus and concentrate makes sense. The amino acid tyrosine and B complex VITAMINS help to produce these two brain chemicals. Dopamine is the pleasure neurotransmitter in the reward centre in the brain. Dopamine is released by neurons into the synapse or gap as a chemical messenger. DRUGS such as marijuana and cocaine interfere with this messaging, affecting the levels of dopamine by trapping it in the synapse, causing euphoria. Schizophrenics and psychotics have very high levels of dopamine. Ten percent of people who try cannabis or hash will become addicted. Cannabis can adversely affect and damage the amygdala in the brain, which links to feelings and emotions.

The 'feel good' endorphins are brain chemicals activated by EXERCISE, so before you reach for the ALCOHOL, or consider anti depressants, get out walking with a friend.

If I need to focus and concentrate on a task and I'm at home and procrastinating I put 10 drops of Basil and Rosemary combined in an oil burner or my bath. Before I go out I use a drop of each in a teaspoon of Jojoba oil on my face and chest to refresh me and wake me up. ESSENTIAL OILS work through the limbic system in the brain which is ancient and linked to aromas and memory. They are also absorbed through the blood capillaries into your body after about an hour. These particular oils are cephalics so they are linked to mind and brain and are stimulating and uplifting.

The Olfactory nerve (aromas) links in to the Limbic system which controls libido, appetite, attitude, emotional states, motivation and sleep cycles. If this area is unbalanced or unstable there may be excessive moodiness and irritation. ESSENTIAL OILS work either as stimulators, relaxants or adaptogens or rebalancers and are an ALTERNATIVE to other pharmaceutical approaches if used with diet, supplements, restorative YOGA and exercise.

St John's Wort is an effective aid for depression but should not be taken with certain medications, so check online or with your doctor. I have also found a supplement called Rhodiola to be helpful as a restabiliser.

"Neuroscientists suggest that the limbic system needs to be kept cool and underactive for us to feel emotionally stable. Studies have shown that the deep limbic system becomes more active and inflamed during women's hormonal cycles. This time of over activity is associated with depression and anxiety."

"Insight Yoga" Sarah Powers*

There are supplements to help if you need to be sharp, focused and to concentrate. Gingko Biloba stimulates blood flow to the brain. It's important to take ANTI OXIDANTS to slow the downward spiral of brain function if we neglect ourselves. The enzyme protein Kinase C is an indicator of brain function that declines rapidly as we age. A brisk walk for forty minutes, a few times a week will slow ageing, as studies on humans show enzyme activity is maintained not lowered.

5-HTP is a supplement that links into serotonin the contentment neurotransmitter which is needed to make the HORMONE melatonin. 5- HTP is from the seeds of Griffonia simplicifolia.

EXERCISE will also help prevent the dopamine receptors in the striatal cortex declining and adversely affecting memory and brain function. The more dopamine we produce the better we feel. It's only recently come to light that exercise positively benefits mental health and brain cells. Stress will ultimately affect your short and long term memory and your ability to make decisions. If you are physically and mentally tired it will lead to difficulties concentrating and you may become impulsive and irritable.

Follow the suggestions under the chapter on SLEEP and find out how and what makes you relax, aside from ALCOHOL and three hours of TV before bed.

The hypothalamus is a collection of nerve cells just above the roof of your mouth which controls and connects to the autonomic nervous system, the hormonal endocrine system and the brain's reward system. The adrenalin "fight or flight" response initialises here as does the message that you're thirsty or hungry and importantly for the survival of the species; the urge for sex. During prolonged periods of stress when the "fight or flight" adrenal response is not turned off, we produce more of the HORMONE cortisol. As well as weight gain around your middle this can cause eye strain, blurred vision and constriction of blood flow to the face.

Mental stress shrinks your brain! It's been shown to adversely affect the anterior cingulated cortex in the brain on MRI scans. The cerebellum in your brain deals with sorting information which may become impaired when very stressed.

The parasympathetic nervous system relaxes us and I regularly use a YOGA posture called Viparit Karani to stimulate and encourage this 'switch off'. Lie on your back with your legs up the wall then lift your hips and place a folded blanket under your mid back so that the buttocks descend. This inverted posture has a positive physiological response in the body and should be held for at least ten minutes.

It's not yet known what causes Alzheimer's disease but it could be linked to heavy metals such as iron, mercury and aluminium so eat fermented vegetables and foods such as Natto and tempeh which is fermented soya and kafir, fermented milk. These fermented foods help to clear heavy metals from the body. Mercury fillings need to be removed by a specialist so that this toxin doesn't enter your system. Alzheimer's will manifest in a variety of ways depending on the area of the brain that's affected. Generally, there's memory loss and confusion as emotional connection and intellect decline.

In *Michal Colgan's* excellent book"*Hormonal Health*"*, he mentions the supplement, acetyl-l-carnitine for optimal brain function and improvement in cognition for people dealing with Alzheimer's disease. Acetyl-l-tyrosine heightens cognitive function as it crosses the blood brain barrier. Take choline as a supplement to maintain brain cell membranes.

New research on Alzheimer's points to viral or bacterial infections affecting the brain. Research is ongoing in regard to treatments and pharmaceutical drugs. I take a turmeric supplement every day as this contains curcumin and lowers inflammation and infection in the body. I have friends who take bee propolis daily to enhance health. Read the chapter HERBS for alternative support.

It's thought that Parkinson's disease, where there is loss of movement, is caused by a drop in Dopamine producing cells in the brain. Take a probiotic and acidophilus regularly to counter heavy metals in your system and to repopulate your BOWEL with beneficial flora. They are chelators so will remove heavy metals. The belief that the bowel is our 'second' brain is gaining in credibility. Go to your health food shop for acidophilus and rhamonus which are essential, healthy bacteria to repopulate your bowels after antibiotics and to maintain good health via the lymphatic system.

Research has shown that common bacteria and spirochete are evident in the central nervous system of Alzheimer's patients but not in people who weren't suffering from it. Alzheimer's patients have high levels of amyloid-beta protein which actually has antibacterial properties. It's being debated that as the damaged brain cells produce more amyloid-beta protein to counter the infection, the deposits of it begin to adversely affect communication, cognition and brain function.

Studies made on the bacteria Borrelia burgdorfei, which causes Lyme's disease and leads to fatigue and flu like symptoms, suggest it enters the brain and forms plaques along the cerebral cortex on the surface of the brain. The infection then worsens, affecting brain tissue and cells. Macrophages in our immune system in our brains normally engulf anything foreign but are unable to, as they become trapped and inefficient within the spirochete plaque. Anti biotics are used effectively against Lyme's disease, which can seem similar to M.E or chronic fatigue. If you want to be checked thoroughly there are companies who can test you for Lyme's.

Recent research has also shown that Curcumin in the spice Turmeric assists the brain macrophages in engulfing bacteria. Amazingly, Curcumin, which can be taken as a supplement can bind to amyloid-beta plaques which ultimately leads to the immune system destroying the bacteria. Curcumin is the polyphenol in Turmeric and is a neuroprotective substance and acts as an ANTI OXIDANT against degeneration, increasing glutathione (which is a powerful antioxidant) production in the brain. Curcumin could be effective in counterbalancing the effects of Fluoride.

Studies are showing that Fluoride, which is added to our water supplies and which we have no choice or say over, is in fact damaging to health. Some countries have banned it and removed it from their water supply. It's now believed to adversely affect the cells of the hippocampus and cerebral cortex in the brain, to lower IQ and to contribute to calcification of the pineal gland.

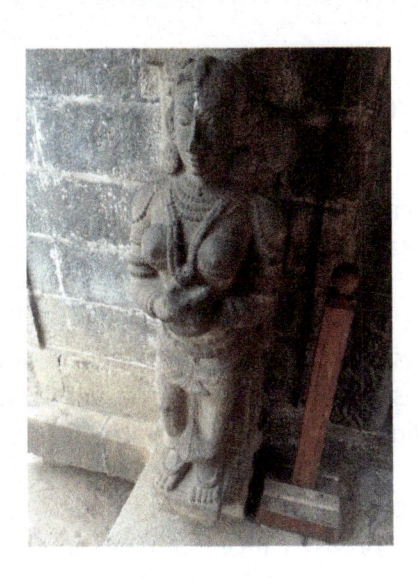

BREASTS

Teach your daughters to examine their breasts every month so that it becomes a habit and part of their routine. Inform them that breast tissue can change and that they can feel swollen or tender before a period, but that any unusual changes should be noted. Prevention and detection saves lives. Lifestyle choices and genetics can impact whether you develop breast cancer later in life.

The main changes to look out for are; changes in the size or shape of the breast, swelling, scaly areas, an "orange peel" appearance or dimpling, a retracted or in-turned nipple and nipple discharge, prominent veins, discomfort and swelling under the armpit in the lymph nodes, lumps in the breast and extreme weight loss.

Lift your arms in front of a mirror to check your breasts. Early on, become familiar with how they look and feel. You can also check them by lying on your back, placing an arm behind your head and using your fingertips, press gently over the breast, starting at the nipple and circling outwards.

Your breasts may be more tender or painful before a period or during MENOPAUSE and they might feel lumpy. 70% of us have fibrocystic breasts with these symptoms (small lumps) and it may be linked to high levels of oestrogen. These can be very uncomfortable and unnerving, but nothing to worry about.

Most lumps you find will be harmless and common. If you are concerned, go to your doctor for a physical examination. Breast cancer can be hereditary. If your female relatives died of it you may have to make difficult choices and to talk to your daughters about it. If you carry the gene mutation BRCA1/2 your specialist will inform you of options. Request an alternative to a mammogram if breast cancer is prevalent in your family, as it's known from recent research that successive and regular mammograms worsen your chances of survival due to the radiation emitted from mammograms.

The medical industry has used mammograms for decades as a diagnostic tool for breast cancer. Almost half of us may have dense breast tissue which means that mammograms won't show abnormal changes. Research over a long period with thousands of women now indicates that having a mammogram does not ensure early detection of life threatening tumours. The research indicates that over-diagnosis has been a problem. Women have then sometimes been subjected to unnecessary surgery and invasive treatment, that wasn't essential for their health and survival. This report from the New York Times states:

"One in five cancers found with mammography and treated was not a threat to the women's health and did not need treatment such as chemotherapy, surgery, or radiation."

In September 1994 the US Journal of the National Cancer Institute published a study showing that women who exercised for four hours a week had a 58% lower risk of breast cancer. If you EXERCISE for between one and three hours a week you'll have a 30% lower risk. Excess levels of oestrogen are implicated in breast cancer and exercise may modify and regulate these hormonal levels.

Consider whether you could navigate the MENOPAUSE without HRT, as it may be linked to breast cancer. Studies show that the risk increases by 15% to 30% after ten years of oestrogen therapy. If you take HRT for more than five years you double your risk of breast cancer (Stanford University in California research study). Within a year of stopping HRT the chances of developing breast cancer had dropped significantly.

We also inadvertently consume or come into contact with xenoestrogens (foreign oestrogens) on a daily basis. Read the chapters on TOXINS, CHEMICALS and PRODUCTS so you're informed about choices and what to avoid. Bisphenol A is a by-product of the plastics industry and has oestrogenic effects on humans.

Oestrogen helps to build the lining of the UTERUS, or womb to embed a fertilised egg in the initial stages of pregnancy. Increased cell growth can lead to cancer and many compounds that we come into contact with play havoc with appropriate levels of hormones for health. These chemical and environmental factors may be triggers for breast cancer. Keep your home as chemical free as possible, have house plants and maintain a constant flow of fresh air by having windows open. Cancer thrives in areas of low oxygen. Avoid drinking from, storing and cooking food in plastic containers. Never leave a plastic bottle full of water in your car then drink from it, as you will ingest harmful chemicals into your system that are now known to be factors in breast cancer development.

If you've been diagnosed with breast cancer you will need to avoid unfermented soy as it's high in phytoestrogens and may cause an increase in the amount of breast cancer cells. Some ESSENTIAL OILS such as fennel, geranium and clary sage should also be avoided at this time, as they are oestrogenic.

This subject is sensitive as most of us grew up with mothers who would never challenge a doctor about mammograms or medication and would follow medical advice to the letter. Opt for a physical examination by a professional if you are concerned about changes in your breasts. Magnetic resonance imaging is a non- ionizing radiation imaging technique used to investigate the possibility of breast cancer and is an alternative to having a mammogram. Research now shows that the incidence of cancer increases in correlation to the number of mammograms you've been subjected to.

A healthy diet and regular, moderate exercise will decrease your chances of facing breast cancer. Read the chapters on VEGETABLES and eat a colourful range and variety of them daily. Avoid excess sugar, processed foods, trans fats, processed fructose, alcohol and fizzy, carbonated soda and drinks. Cancer feeds on SUGAR.

There may be a link to saturated fat and breast cancer so cut down on dairy milk and red meat. Limit cheese consumption but have a small amount of good quality, hard cheese once a week. Avoid processed oils and margarine and use a small amount of butter

BREASTS

or coconut oil instead. If you're overweight, your fatty tissue can retain toxic waste and toxins will be stored in breast tissue. There are also a lot of antibiotics, growth hormones and CHEMICALS in most farmed animals, which you need to avoid. Eat unsaturated fat in pumpkin and sesame seeds with a small handful of NUTS and olive oil as a salad dressing, as these are beneficial for optimal health.

Take a quality multi vitamin and mineral supplement and a curcumin supplement, taken from the spice turmeric, for optimal breast health. Try to expose your SKIN to the sun for a healthy dose of vitamin D. Vitamin D will reduce your chances of dealing with breast cancer as it aids your body on a cellular level to fight cancer. Take 40 ng/ml of vitamin D with vitamin K2 if you're taking a supplement.

To ensure you eat enough vitamin A, another cancer buster, buy organic, free range eggs. Eat fermented vegetables such as sauerkraut, take a probiotic with acidophilus to ensure a healthy BOWEL and optimally functioning immune system. Fibre is essential for good health as soluble fibre binds to excess oestrogen, so that the body can excrete it efficiently. If you don't have enough fibre from fruit and vegetables and are regularly constipated you may have painful, lumpy, fibrocystic breasts. When you have a bowel movement your system removes waste, toxins and used hormones. Old oestrogen needs to leave your body so that it's not recycled around your system again.

If you're planning a pregnancy or have friends and family who are, advise them to breast feed if possible, as there is a powerful link to growth, healthy BOWELS and BRAIN development when a child is breast fed as opposed to formula products. There is a combination of factors and nutrients in breast milk that cannot be mimicked.

If you are debating whether or not to have breast implants, research it fully before you decide. Go online and read the stories about women who've had them. It might be true that you'll feel more confident, and that your body image and self esteem will be heightened. The risks are high. Having breast implants can be hazardous and detrimental to your health. A large percentage of breast augmentation operations will result in silicone leakage from rupture and infections. You may also experience 'capsular contracture' where scar tissue causes the implant to feel painful and solid, not soft. How old are you now? If you're contemplating it in your twenties you could affect a future baby's health. Bear in mind that after just twelve years fifty percent of women will have leaky implants and after twenty five years, two thirds of them. That means that silicone could migrate to your organs and systems. If you opt for saline implants, bacteria and fungus can multiply in and around the implant. There is also a chance of developing a rare type of non Hodgkin's lymphoma cancer. Take time to really think about the repercussions.

Wear comfortable, unrestricting, unwired bras when you can, so that the lymph fluid can flow in the top of your body. Our lymphatic systems filter toxins from our bodies. Don't ever sleep in your bra and try not to wear one longer than ten hours.

Extreme stress and shock are known to be triggers for cancer. Research and studies have shown that the death of a partner, child, or loss of a valued career or divorce were factors in breast cancer. Those women who

BREASTS

expressed their anguish openly were more likely to cope and survive.

Take time to go to a weekly YOGA, QIGONG or MEDITATION and relaxation class so that you find some peace and quiet time. If you have been diagnosed with breast cancer, your own practise of these past-times will be very helpful and beneficial. It may be a difficult, challenging time to practise positivity but more women are surviving after breast cancer and hopefully, new drugs will be available in the coming years that are affordable.

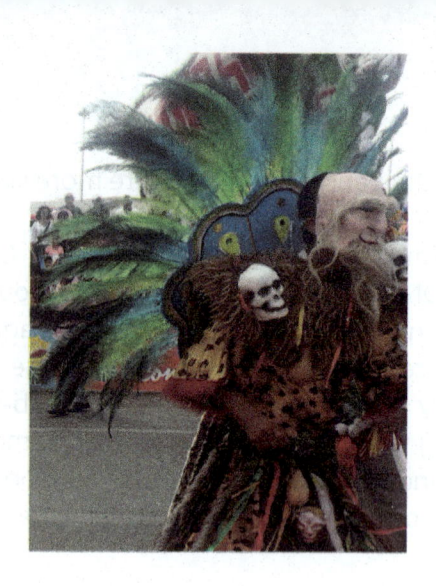

CHEMICALS

Make sure you open your windows to air your living space as there are so many chemicals from personal care, cleaning and decorating products. The combined effect of these is unknown, but the human body carries a cocktail of chemicals that are not conducive for optimal health. Good reasons to let the fresh air in are; cancer thrives on a lack of oxygen and if condensation builds and your living space becomes damp and mouldy, this will adversely affect your lungs and cardiovascular system. If your immune system is working overtime it has less chance of doing its job efficiently.

Have houseplants in your space as they remove toxins from the air. Don't use synthetic air fresheners, use an aromatherapy oil burner. (Always blow candles out before you leave). You can buy an electric ESSENTIAL OIL burner if you have small children or pets. Keep dust to a minimum as chemicals and mites accumulate in house dust.

CHEMICALS

I use baking powder, salt and vinegar mixed with lemon juice as a household cleaner as I find my eyes streaming if I use certain products. The company Ecover has a range of natural products for washing dishes and clothes.

Natural ingredients are in abundance and cost very little, if you're thinking about making your own personal care PRODUCTS. The Environmental Working Group's Skin Deep database will give you information about chemical free products. Yes, they can be more expensive but you're assisting the planet and maintaining your long term health.

Flame retardant chemicals are hazardous to health and unfortunately are in cushions, mattresses and carpeting. If you can, use wool or silk products and opt for a 'green' alternative.

Here are some of the chemicals to avoid. Start reading the labels on the back of products:

BISPHENOL A

This chemical is a by product of the plastics industry and is known to produce oestrogenic effects in humans. Your food may be wrapped in this plastic and a residue of it will be left in the food. I try to buy fruit and vegetables from markets once a week and ask for brown paper bags that I can recycle.

PARABENS

A synthetic form of Parabens derived from petrochemicals is used in cosmetics. Parabens easily penetrate the SKIN, which absorbs seventy percent of what we put on it. This is a weekly chemical cocktail which we inadvertently, slowly damage our health with. Parabens are found in many products such as shampoos, conditioners and shower gels. Get into the habit of looking on the back of products you buy. Related chemicals to avoid are methylparaben, butylparaben, propylparaben , isobutylparaben and ethylparaben.

Parabens are now known to interfere with normal HORMONE function as they mimic oestrogen, the main female hormone and have been linked to human BREAST cancer. They may also affect the male reproductive system. Studies have also shown that methylparaben on the skin reacts with UVB, ages skin and accelerates DNA damage. Propyl paraben is used as a food preservative in cakes and food dyes.

If you look at ways to reduce your weekly spending by checking comparison websites for bills, taking a packed lunch or reducing the twice daily bought cappuccinos then you can afford quality products. Some companies strive to obtain organic ingredients and to reduce chemicals and these are more expensive. It's worth it as the long list of chemicals in most products can have an insidious, long term affect on your wellbeing. Start checking labels and then try to make your own cleaning products adding ESSENTIAL OILS such as tea tree, clove or eucalyptus for an anti bacterial action.

DIETHANOLAMINE

Cocamide and lauramide are used in creamy, foaming products such as soaps, cleansers and shampoos. DEA (Diethanolamine) is found in sunscreens and moisturisers. High doses of these over prolonged periods are linked to precancerous changes in skin and thyroid and liver function. If DEA reacts with nitrates in cosmetics they form nitrosamines, a possible human carcinogen. The European Union Cosmetics Directive restricts the concentration of Cocamide and Lauramide DEA in products.

DIBUTYL PHTHALATE

This is used in nail products and dyes as a plasticizer. It is also used in fragrance. Don't use nail varnish or perfume during pregnancy. It is a suspected hormone endocrine disrupter and may impair FERTILITY or damage the foetus.

SODIUM LAURETH SULPHATE

SLES (Sodium Laureth Sulphate) is a chemical used in detergents and products such as shampoo to make it foamy. It may be contaminated with ethylene oxide and 1-4 dioxin. The first of these is a known cause of cancer in humans and can also damage the nervous system. It may interfere with normal human development.

PETROLEUM

Mineral oil jelly can be contaminated with polycyclic aromatic hydro carbons (PAH's) and is associated with cancer, skin irritation and allergies. Buy Burts bee's balm not Vaseline for your dry lips.

TRICLOSAN

Triclocarban is added to products such as deodorants and toothpastes to prevent bacterial contamination but has chemical properties similar to some pesticides and pharmaceuticals. Check labels on kitchenware, clothing and furniture for this hormone endocrine disruptor. Recent studies show that Triclosan alters hormone regulation and has been found in urine in studies. It's known to accumulate in the liver and fatty tissue in the body. In cultures of breast cancer it had an oestrogen like effect on the proliferation of cancer cells. Remember that your body absorbs 70% of what you put on your skin. Before you buy a deodorant check the label for Aluminium (which has also been linked to breast cancer) and Triclosan and don't buy it. There are effective, natural plant alternatives which are sold in health shops. I'm enjoying using one by Jason under my armpits at the moment.

PHENOXYETHANOL

Baby wipes and Pampers can contain this chemical which could be toxic for the liver and blood so check labels.

Polyethylene glycols (PEG compounds) are petroleum based and used in solvents, softeners and moisture carriers. It is also found in pharmaceutical laxatives. This chemical can be contaminated with ethylene oxide and 1,4-dioxane. Propylene glycol is a related chemical and both function as penetration enhancers, allowing toxic additives to be absorbed more readily through your SKIN and into your organs and systems.

CHEMICALS

PHENYLENEDIAMINE

This chemical is in coal tar dyes and may be contaminated with heavy metals which could be detrimental to the BRAIN and optimal health. Check the packet for CI followed by a five digit number. A friend has recently suggested using the hair colourant tintsofnature.com for a less toxic way to dye your hair.

It takes time and diligence to clean up your life in regard to minimising toxic overload so take small steps in any way you can.

CHI

Ancient Hindu Yogic, Asian and Oriental Chinese philosophies have long offered the belief that a primordial energy and life force known as prana, chi, ki, qi or lung in Tibetan, underpins and permeates the Universe and animates us all. The physical, material world, everything organic and inorganic, the Earth and all living, breathing beings are revitalised and maintained from this source.

These ancient, knowing civilisations postulated that this life force runs through meridians or invisible pathways perhaps intertwined with fascia and connective tissue in the material body, and used during acupuncture in Chinese healing and medicine. In the Indian Yogic system the prana runs through thousands of Nadis or "energy tubes". These are no longer just theory, but based on scientific investigation. They are a factor in optimal health, which is why acupuncture and massage forms, like Tui na, alleviate symptoms and help clear conditions and increase energy.

Mind, movement, intention and breath influence and move Chi. The meridians link and interconnect the flow of energy through systems and organs in our bodies maintaining balance and vitality. This Chi may become polluted or stagnant and distorted so affecting our mobility, positivity and overall health.

CHI

Chi is constantly being absorbed, used and emitted as a source from the infinite or Divine but is neither created or destroyed.

"It is only by Qi that the planets move, the sun shines, the wind blows, the elements exist, and human beings live and breathe. It is the cohesion of the body mind spirit and the integration of the myriad aspects of each individual human being. It is spoken of with reverence because it is the basis of life and when gone awry, the basis of disease."

Dianne M. Connelly Traditional Acupuncture.*

CHOCOLATE

Eating dark chocolate in moderation is good for your health. A few small squares a day of 70 to 80% cacao will benefit you, as it's now known to be full of ANTIOXIDANTS and probiotics with anti-inflammatory effects. Cacao powder is high in IRON, calcium and magnesium. The body's 'good' bacteria in the lower digestive system breaks down the chocolate so that the anti inflammatory compounds can easily be absorbed and utilised by your body.

If you take care of your gut and BOWEL health you will be healthier overall, as it's now believed to be an important area that if problematic, can lead to disease. The antioxidants in chocolate, polyphenols, assist your immune system and certain compounds act to relax your blood vessels so benefitting your cardiovascular system and heart.

The fibre in cocoa is also broken down into short fatty acid chains which are beneficial. Chocolate is satisfying and comforting. This doesn't apply to the cheap candy and milk chocolate which is full of sugar and has no nutritional value.

Chocolate in its pure form as Cacao seeds is turned into cocoa after it's been roasted and as it's naturally bitter, some form of SUGAR is added. Check the form of the sugar so that you avoid fructose. There are many

CHOCOLATE

excellent fair trade products on the market now so enjoy and savour a mouthful every day.

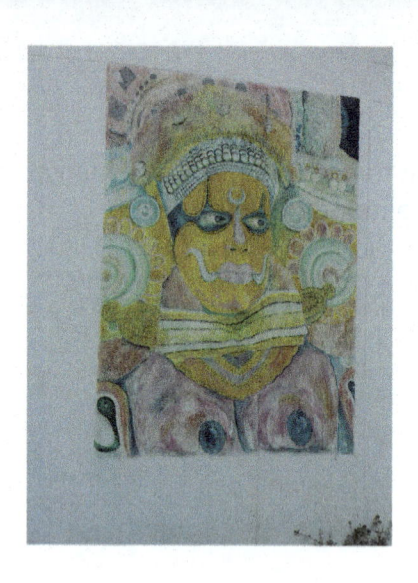

CHLAMYDIA

Chlamydia is a sexually transmitted disease caused by a type of bacteria, Chlamydia trachomatis. It's the most common STI. The under twenty five age group seem to contract it more than any other. You may be unaware that you have it until a few weeks after you've had sex with an infected partner. Symptoms of Chlamydia include; yellow or green vaginal discharge, traces of blood in your urine or from the back passage or anus, needing to urinate more often and feeling discomfort when you do. Penetrative sex may be painful (dyspareunia). You may have pelvic or abdominal pain.

If you contract Chlamydia there's a possibility that it could damage your fallopian tubes (the connection between the OVARIES and womb or UTERUS). This could lead to pelvic inflammatory disease (PID) which is a serious condition and causes pelvic and abdominal pain.

If there is scarring or damage in a fallopian tube, the egg (ova) that's released from the ovary and travels

CHLAMYDIA

down the fallopian tube to the womb, may be blocked or hindered. There's more risk of having an ectopic pregnancy, where the egg is fertilised and starts to develop in the fallopian tube instead of the uterus, if you have Chlamydia. The probability of infertility is higher.

If you do fall pregnant and don't treat Chlamydia, you have a higher risk of a premature birth. You may be offered a caesarean birth, but if not, your child could be born with an eye infection or pneumonia, as it may come into contact with the Chlamydia bacteria as it passes down the birth canal.

Chlamydia is treated with four antibiotic tablets. It's really important to go to a health food shop to buy acidophilus and a probiotic after antibiotics. Take the probiotics for a couple of months as antibiotics destroy the good, beneficial bacteria in the BOWEL.

Insist that your new partner wears a condom to lessen the chance of contracting a sexually transmitted disease, some of which can be initially treated, but not cured. Herpes 2 is a virus which causes very painful blisters around the genital area and can be passed to a partner through penetrative SEX or oral sex. Herpes 1 causes cold sores around the mouth area and most of us have this in our systems by the time we are twenty. Avoid kissing or giving oral sex if you have a cold sore.

The initial signs you may have genital herpes are; redness and swelling in the area, pain while urinating, tingling or itching around the genitals. Painful blisters will become evident and are contagious as they contain the virus. They will dry and heal over after awhile but avoid having sex for a week after this.

Although you'll be given medication to ease the discomfort of genital herpes, there may be recurring outbreaks if you become stressed or tired. If you have been diagnosed or feel you are about to have an outbreak, rest, by getting some early nights, avoid thongs and tights and nylon underwear and drink plenty of water. If you can, have a few days where you don't wear pants at all or wear loose cotton, bamboo or hemp underwear.

Anti viral medications can be prescribed to lessen symptoms and prevent a full breakout, but they won't cure it. Your doctor may give you famciclovir (famvir), acyclovir (zocirax) or valacyclovir (valtrex). Try to avoid taking acetaminophen(Tylenol) or aspirin in excess for the discomfort and pain, as these are known to disrupt the brain and stomach lining and cause nausea and kidney problems. Only take paracetamol and pain killers when you really need to, as it takes the liver many hours to process them.

If you discover you have herpes or have an outbreak, sprinkle baking soda on the area if you have some and steep a chamomile teabag in hot water for five minutes. Once it's cooled put the teabag in the fridge for ten minutes, add a teaspoonful of apple cider vinegar and a drop of tea tree, then place it over the blistered area to reduce pain and swelling. In extreme cases, use an icepack placed over a flannel.

There are natural herbal alternatives to ease the discomfort of genital herpes. Taking a bath with ESSENTIAL OILS cools and calms the area and reduces inflammation. Put five drops of tea tree and five of lavender in a teaspoonful of coconut or jojoba oil. Pour this under a running tap and soak in a warm bath for twenty minutes. Aloe Vera as a gel is cooling and healing too. As supplements, Echinacea and zinc boost the immune system. Take lysine tablets to prevent further herpes outbreaks. Echinacea can also be applied as an ointment on the infected area. Propolis, a bee product has also had results as a cream to apply to blisters. Always wash your hands thoroughly afterwards. Consult a homeopath if you decide to treat herpes with homeopathy.

However difficult or challenging it feels, you must tell a regular partner or a new lover that you have herpes and they will then decide if they want to go ahead with the relationship. Wearing condoms lessens the risk of contracting or passing genital herpes on.

The incidences of gonorrhoea have recently increased. There was a 53% increase in cases between 2012 and 2015. It used to be known as "The Clap". You might not show symptoms but could have green or yellow discharge and pain when urinating. The latest news on this STI is that some strains of gonorrhoea are now resistant to antibiotics. It's treated with an injection and a tablet.

Syphilis cases increased 75% in the same period. HIV may be unthinkable, but when you sleep with someone for the first time, you have no knowledge of their previous partners and their health. HIV is the virus that can lead to AIDS. Wear a condom until you've both had a complete check up.

The symptoms of Chlamydia are different in men. If your partner has conjunctivitis, along with a sore throat and a white, yellow or green discharge from his penis tell him to go to his doctor to be checked for it. One or both testicles may have swelled and it could be painful to urinate. It may also lead to the infection spreading to the prostate gland and to lower back pain.

The decision in the heat of the moment to have sex without a condom, before you know the partner, may have long term repercussions which affect your life deeply. Teenage pregnancies are high in Britain. If you fall pregnant you then have the emotional task of deciding whether to have a termination or abortion. There may be deep regret or guilt later in life, particularly if you find you are unable to conceive in your late thirties or early forties when your chances of a healthy pregnancy decrease.

If you feel that it would potentially ruin a promising career or university dream that you've set your heart on, or if you already have a few children and it's come as an unexpected surprise in your early forties, talk to someone who can advise you about termination.

Most abortions are performed within the first fourteen weeks. You could be offered one up to twenty weeks. If you are a staunch Catholic or have strong prolife opinions, abortion will not be an option for you. When does life begin? You can fall pregnant in your late forties if you're still having periods sporadically, due to the onset of menopause, but the chances are low.

A test where the nuccal folds are assessed or placental fluid tested can ascertain if you are carrying a child with Downes syndrome. This can be a rewarding, deeply loving child, but a challenging situation depending on the degree the child has it. These people tend to pass away at a younger age but can have a fulfilling life. Research this if you've fallen pregnant and both you and your partner are over thirty five, when the chances of having a Downes syndrome child increase.

Think carefully before you decide about a termination and once you've made your mind up have someone

CHLAMYDIA

waiting for you, whether they are family or friend so that you have support afterwards. Trust that after weighing everything up, you've made the right decision for you. Condoms are slightly awkward, and the sensation might not be the same during intercourse, but if it prevents you from suffering a sexually transmitted disease or unwanted pregnancy, then it's worth using one. If you have had sex without one, the morning after pill is also an option, but not something you want to be taking regularly. Read the chapter on CONTRACEPTIVES for other options regarding avoiding pregnancy.

COCONUT MILK AND OIL

Coconut milk is rich in magnesium, iron, potassium and the ANTIOXIDANTS vitamins B, C and E. Use it sparingly in smoothies, (don't overdo the fruit because of the fructose which is just another form of sugar) soups and curries to enhance the taste. It will give your meal a creamier texture whilst boosting your health. It will also discourage candida albican yeast, viruses including HIV and herpes, bacteria and giardia lamblia. These pathogens can cause misery and discomfort and once lodged and dormant in your body, can cause fatigue and further recurrent infections due to your immune system being undermined. Recent research suggests that if your system is struggling with them and is already compromised, it can pave the way for cancer.

Half of the beneficial healthy 'fat' in coconut oil is Lauric acid which is a medium chain fatty acid which can cross cell membranes and which your liver converts to energy not fat. Your body converts Lauric acid into Monolaurin, a mono glyceride which is the active component to target the pathogens in your body.

Butter and coconut oil are the best choices for cooking so give up margarines, sunflower, soya and canola as they are processed and you are on a path to eliminate most of the pre-packaged processed food from your shopping trolley and life. Frying with vegetable oils

COCONUT MILK AND OIL

means they oxidise and may cause extreme inflammation in your body leading to degenerative diseases such as Alzheimer's and heart disease. Look at the labels on food you buy and avoid transfat and cane sugar for the same reason. If you don't cook then take a coconut oil supplement, as it is a super food!

It's challenging to avoid palm oil as it's in a myriad of forms in so many products and foodstuffs, but it has wrecked havoc and its harvesting has resulted in the clearing and decimation of rain forests in Asia. This means that orang-utans and native species lose their homes and that ultimately our eco systems are adversely affected. Carbon dioxide levels change and weather will become freakier if we continue along the path of clearing trees to make big bucks. Sign any petitions you see in regard to this and make it known you don't want the negative effects of palm oil on your conscience or in your life.

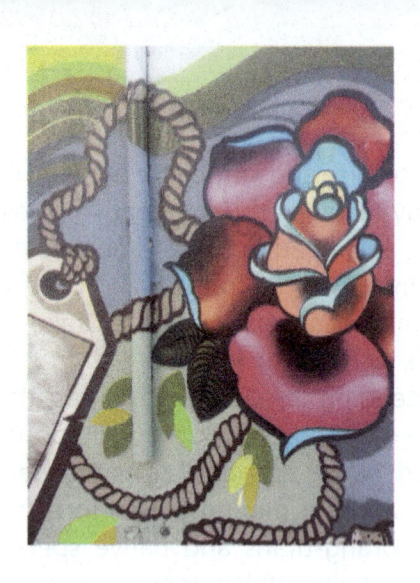

CONTRACEPTIVES

Unplanned pregnancies can cause a myriad of emotions. If you decide the timing's terrible you're faced with options which may have repercussions years later, but at the time are feasible and rational. If you're reading this and you're eighteen think carefully about your actions and decide how you feel about having children. Your thoughts may change in the following decade.

It's become very common for women to put off having children because of excellent, well paid jobs and fulfilling careers, leaving it until they are in their late thirties. FERTILITY will take a down turn as early as your late twenties and the chances of IVF treatments turning into a successful pregnancy are very small in your mid forties. You can be surprised by an unplanned pregnancy in your forties too, so consider contraception if you're sure you don't want a child.

Certain sexually transmitted diseases are increasing and the only ways to avoid these are to abstain or use

CONTRACEPTIVES

a condom, however much your one night stand or new partner insists that they don't have anything nasty and detest condoms. There will be times when your spilt second decisions will ripple and reverberate through the rest of your life in ways you cannot imagine, along with physical pain and emotional anguish. Not everything in life can be meticulously planned and carried out but consider your thoughts and feelings without blindly rushing into situations. Once you have contracted the virus genital Herpes, there is no cure and although it abates, you will need to keep a watchful eye on flare-ups.

There are a number of other options regarding contraception aside from condoms and the Pill which you take daily. Sexual drive and libido may drop whilst on the Pill. The combined pill with oestrogen and progesterone is effective one to seven days from taking it. If you miss a day or have diarrhoea or vomiting you can fall pregnant. The mini pill only contains progestogen without oestrogen. If you are over thirty and a heavy smoker this may be prescribed for you. You have to take it in the same three hour period every day.

LARC (long acting reversible contraception) offers long term protection but if you stop taking them, normal levels of hormones resume.

If you don't mind injections, this method lasts from eight to thirteen weeks, but there may be a delay of around a year before HORMONE levels return to normal. It uses progesterone to prevent pregnancy and is a quick, easy option.

The ultra-Uterine device or IUS is a small, plastic device which is placed in the womb and releases a lower daily dose of the hormone progestogen which prevents pregnancy. It thickens the mucous at the top of the vagina at the cervix. It can work for three to five years and is an option if you have heavy periods as they can lessen after six months.

The subdermal plant is put in your arm and releases progestogen. Bleeding can be irregular using this method, but fertility will resume straight away after it's removed. It can be quickly removed by a nurse. This implant is an option for women who can't have oestrogen.

The IUD (intrauterine device) or copper coil also returns hormone levels to normal when removed and can be placed in the womb for five to ten years. It can be painful to insert.

DEBT

There are many jobs on offer today that require a degree. You'll have to weigh up whether you want to devote a few years to full time study or if you're ready to apply for jobs. Not everyone is academic. Look at vocational courses in technical colleges or an apprenticeship in something that interests you.

If your 'A' level grades were high and you know what you want to study, start thinking about options and where you want to go.

If you're planning to go to university or thinking of sending your daughter, you'll need to think seriously about the costs. There are two parts to student finance. The first part is the Tuition Fee Loan which is a loan from the government. Most courses at university are £9,000 (at time of writing October 2016). As some universities have higher ranking in regard to the quality of lecturers and courses, some courses will be more expensive. The government allows universities to charge more if they decide to. This tuition fee loan is transferred from the government to the university, so won't show up on your bank statement.

The second part of finance is your Maintenance Loan which will be paid into your bank account. Discuss whether you would like to live in Halls, or stay at home, or share a house or flat with a group. Your budget will have to be concise, depending on where you have decided to live or if you are travelling in to university daily. The loan will need to cover your social life and food as well as accommodation. The amount of money your parents make as a wage will also factor into this. There are other grants, bursaries or scholarships for low income families. This maintenance loan will be paid into your account in three instalments over the academic year.

This could help you to budget. https://www.ucas.com/ucas/undergraduate/finance-and-support/budget-calculator

Once you have finished the university course and are earning over £21,000 a year you start paying the loan back to the government. The loan is based on 9% of your annual income. If you're earning £25,000, you'll be paying £30 a month. Interest rate while studying is inflation, plus 3%. If you change jobs and earn less than £21,000, the repayments stop. This debt does not affect your credit rating or applications for mortgages, loans and credit cards. After thirty years the debt is cancelled, no matter how much you paid back.

Be very careful with how you use credit cards. Unfortunately, many people these days have no choice but to resort to using one for emergencies. Due to wages and the cost of living they might not have been able to save so live from month to month. Your credit rating will show a low score if you do not make payments over a period of time. This will be detrimental the next time you apply for a mortgage, loan or overdraft.

If you have decide to go self employed have some savings behind you, as debt can spiral out of control if the cash flow in to the business doesn't match your essential outgoings and you're paying a chunk of your

DEBT

wage to a business loan. However, sometimes you need to speculate to accumulate, and a loan, if managed well could give you the necessary means to start a fulfilling, successful business. More and more people will work part time or have a few different jobs. Have a budget with your ingoings and outgoings, so it's transparent and you can see if you are living beyond your means.

Our society started to revere material gains and bling in the eighties when greed was seen as ambition and cash as power. Don't feel you have to compete with other people's jewellery or cars or furniture, clothes and shoes. These things are superficial and might not bring you deep, long lasting joy. There's a difference between rewarding yourself with things you enjoy in moderation and wanting to brag, compete and show off.

We can all be drawn into slick advertising and marketing. We grew up on it and it's clever and subliminal. If you feel that filling a gap in your life comes from splurging and buying goods with a credit card, you could enjoy the feelings of temporary happiness and pleasure. That feeling will sour if you don't pay off the credit card you used for that brief sense of relief. If you only pay the minimum monthly amount needed on that credit card the interest on it will become a looming figure that you will struggle to completely settle. Debt can escalate over a short period so only use credit cards if you need to.

DETOX DAY

Our bodies are constantly monitoring the effects of pollution, pesticides and anything we put on our skin. Our lungs and skin expel waste and our livers work overtime, especially if we binge drink.

The changing of the seasons is an ideal time to step away from routine and everyday life, so put aside a day when you turn off your mobile and laptop and turn inwards to nurture yourself.

Start the day with a mug of hot water, add a teaspoon of flax or olive oil, some grated ginger, a teaspoon of apple cider vinegar and honey or an alternative to sugar. Add a squeeze of fresh lemon juice. Ginger aids digestion, soothing the stomach, stimulating the liver and contains important MINERALS such as calcium, phosphorous, magnesium and potassium.

Afterwards, use a body bristle brush on dry skin which stimulates the lymphatic system into releasing excess fluid and toxic waste. Invest in a good quality natural bristle brush for this and starting at your hands and feet brush upwards quite vigorously along your limbs, towards your heart. You're brushing towards the main lymphatic drainage points in the armpits, groin and sides of the neck.

Take some time on the buttocks as the circulation is poor here. The triceps can become flabby so focus

DETOX DAY

on them too. Brush under the ribs beginning on your right side over to the left and down to your left hipbone, across the lower abdomen to the right hipbone and back up so you brush to stimulate the BOWEL.

Make a smoothie with pineapple, carrot, a pinch of cinnamon, COCONUT MILK and sip it slowly to aid digestion. Cinnamon stabilises blood sugar levels.

Once that has gone down, treat yourself to a bath. It should be warm, not too hot, with a handful of Epsom salts and some sea salt in it. Epsom salts has beneficial magnesium in it which calms your system. If you prefer a seaweed or mud product check the label for added chemicals before you buy it. ESSENTIAL OILS of juniper, cypress, geranium, peppermint and lavender are ideal to detoxify and rejuvenate as they stimulate the lymphatic system. They will soothe you as you switch off and relax. Only use ten drops in total and blend in a tablespoon of milk, jojoba or grape seed oil before pouring under the running tap. Light some candles and put some soft, quiet music on whilst in the bath and then soak for twenty minutes.

After your bath, relax and read a novel or magazine or practise some QIGONG, YOGA or MEDITATION. Lie down on your bed or mat and placing your hands on your lower belly imagine a large balloon there that you're gradually inflating then slowly deflate this and repeat for ten minutes. This has a powerful, positive effect on your nervous system. Afterwards, scan through your body, imagining that you're melting into the earth as you follow your natural breath for another ten minutes. This increases oxygen intake, balances carbon dioxide and is deeply relaxing. If you've been feeling lethargic, exhausted and burnt out you might want to do this over two or three days or once a week.

Clear your fridge and cupboards of any temptations before the day.

Before you prepare your meal have a large glass of filtered or boiled WATER. Grill, roast or steam some vegetables with garlic in COCONUT oil and eat slowly to aid digestion. Blend green vegetables, beetroot, parsley, cabbage, tomatoes and an onion with garlic, cumin and pepper for a nourishing soup. Beetroot cleanses the liver, kidneys and gall bladder. Add a small amount of cooked brown, not white rice as brown absorbs rubbish from the bowels. White rice is a starchy carbohydrate and a FOOD that's high on the glycaemic index.

During the day drink HERBAL teas such as ginger and lemon, nettle, peppermint, fennel or dandelion with half a teaspoon of manuka honey or luo han kuo, which is a natural sweetener, as this will support the liver and kidneys and sooth your digestive system. Limit your calories for the day so your digestive system gets a much needed rest too. Snack on apples, which are high in pectin. These are cleansing for the BOWEL as is chopped celery or a few blueberries. Have a shot of wheatgrass to aid detoxification and give you a super boost of VITAMIN C and IRON.

Take some time to declutter and clear out old makeup, cosmetics and clothes then put a few drops of sage ESSENTIAL OIL in a burner with water to cleanse the space you live in.

There are supplements to support liver health such as milk thistle (silymarin), which helps boost the levels of glutathione in your body. Glutathione is a powerful ANTIOXIDANT and detoxifier. I occasionally take the

DETOX DAY

HERB goldenseal for a few months too. Patrick Holford's company Higher Nature sell a product called colofibre for a bowel cleanse and Paraclens.

An excellent way to deep cleanse your teeth and gums is to swish either almond, COCONUT, sesame or grape seed oil around in your mouth for ten minutes, using it as a vigorous mouthwash to remove waste, TOXINS and bacteria from between your teeth and gums. It will turn into a milky, white liquid. This will also draw excess catarrh and phlegm from your sinuses. Spit it into a bin not down the sink and make it a weekly habit. Using oil as a mouthwash and to clean between your teeth is an ancient, effective Ayurvedic practise from a healing system in India. Floss your teeth when watching TV or in the bath so you do it regularly. I have suffered as a result of not caring for my teeth and have experienced pain and problems. I use the oil swilling regularly now.

These practises can be used every day. Ensure that you regularly take a day for yourself when you can, to recharge your body and mind and to be still, to focus on just 'being' not 'doing'.

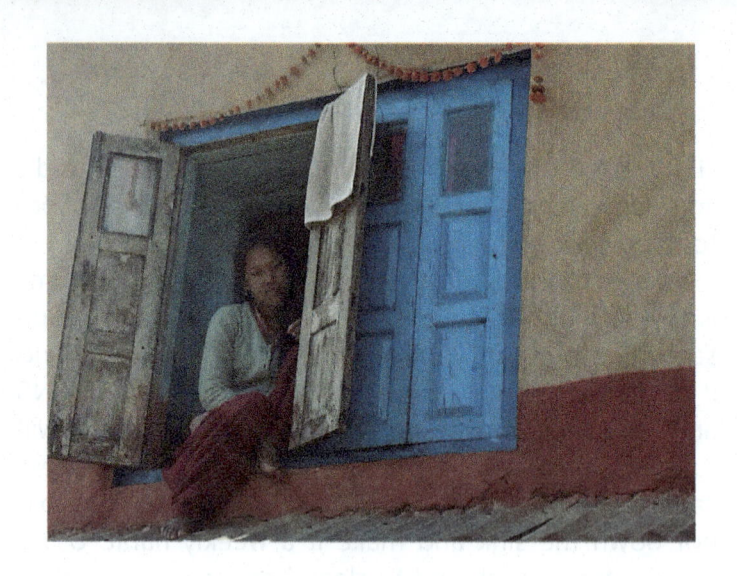

DIARY

Plan exciting events and meetings with friends so your diary has pages of things to look forward to but ensure that occasionally you take a day to be alone, switch off your phone, laptop and the TV and just relax doing nothing very much, just 'being'.

As soon as you wake up write down any dreams, then spend ten minutes writing about how you're feeling generally, any thoughts or emotions that have surfaced so that you're aware of them.

If you're trying to lose weight it's essential that you keep a FOOD diary as we tend to consume more than we think in a day.

Have a section in your diary for the things you felt grateful for, even if they were very simple. GRATITUDE is powerful. Things like a warm smile from your partner or a gesture from a neighbour can brighten your day. There is always something to be thankful for, but we take so many things for granted.

DIARY

Encourage your children to write in a diary every day. I had a five year diary from the age of eight and found it hilarious and life affirming to read back over it as an adult. Small celebrations and ridiculous sulks are part of growing up. Remembering days out with family and friends allows you to revisit memories you may have forgotten about, and it's these days and your relationships, that make life the beautiful, but fragile, short journey it is.

Every day life and those connections and events weave through our days in our diaries.

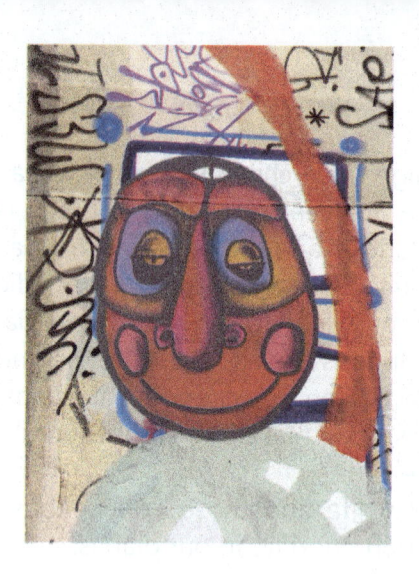

DRUGS

Psychoactive substances (or highs), are not fit for human consumption. They contain substances which produce similar effects to E tablets or Ecstasy, hash, skunk, cannabis or cocaine. Some are sedatives and some stimulants. They may be sold on the street or in 'head shops' under names like snow white, benzo fury, exodus, clockwork orange, ivory wave or spice. Think twice.

Methiopropamine, benzodiazepines and alpha-methyltryptamine are some of the chemical substances in 'highs'. There may be other unknown additives or fillers in drugs.

Mephedrone was one of the first 'highs', and is a stimulant also known as meow meow. Deaths from this drug occurred in 2009 after snorting or injecting it. Going to a music festival is an amazing way to spend a weekend away with friends and there are hundreds of opportunities in Europe and around the world to go. Taking 'highs' and laughing gas has become part of the experience. Deaths related to these drugs have increased dramatically. You might think it will never happen to you or your friends, but it could.

In 2013 there were a hundred and seventy three deaths from 'highs'. You have no idea what is actually in the chemical cocktail you're taking, and if you combine it with ALCOHOL and amphetamines the risks increase. The age of people taking them ranges from fifteen to thirty.

The effects of taking these chemical 'highs' include; feeling paranoid and anxious with panic attacks and having psychotic episodes with seizures and hallucinations. Physically, you may feel nauseous, vomit blood, and experience chest pain and heart palpitations. If you value your life and long term mental health think twice.

In the spring of 2016 the government set up the Psychoactive Substances Act in response to the alarming increase in deaths from these drugs.

Cannabis is also known as hash and marijuana and is smoked with nicotine or in pipes or put in cakes. The active ingredient in hash is tetrahydrocannabinol (THC). There is an ongoing debate about hash due to its effective use as a pain reliever for people who have terminal illness. Our bodies contain receptors for cannabis indicating that it may have been used for millennia.

Interestingly, there is a lot of information on the internet about people with cancer who have been told they don't have long to live, taking resin made from the buds of high quality marijuana plants. Some people's testimonials claim that taking THC shrunk their tumours and saved their lives. This does need to be investigated by scientists in controlled studies.

Hash and skunk, along with barbiturates, mephedrone and amphetamines are class B drugs. They're illegal. People who deal drugs are selfish idiots and the scum of the earth. Their actions ripple out into grief and anguish of family and friends who experience addiction or the death of a loved one. You'll spend and waste a huge amount of money if you allow yourself to become addicted to drugs.

Skunk is a form of marijuana or hash. It is relatively new, and is the result of crossing two cannabis plants. It is much stronger than the pot or hash that was smoked in the sixties and seventies. At that time there was 1.2% THC in hash. Skunk can contain 16.2%. If you already have a history of mental health you can spiral downwards very quickly. There have been reports that teenagers and people in their twenties have developed extreme mental health problems, psychotic episodes and schizophrenia from smoking skunk. If you smoke it you may experience panic attacks and paranoia that occurs beyond the day you take it.

Long term regular use of cannabis can cause depression because THC in hash lowers the contentment neurotransmitter serotonin. It also affects the anterior cingulated cortex in your BRAIN lowering drive, motivation and ambition. Cannabis interferes with the connection and transmission of natural BRAIN chemicals (neurotransmitters).

Your brain has 'plasticity', which means it is capable of expanding and changing and developing new neural pathways. Learning novel, stimulating things develops the brain. When you smoke hash or cannabis, new nerve connections cannot be made. If you're studying for A levels, at college or university or have a challenging job, your memory and concentration levels will be adversely affected. This is due to cannabis damaging the grey matter, hippocampus and prefrontal cortex in your BRAIN which is connected to learning. Ultimately, your grades and achievements will be lower than what you're actually capable of.

If you reach a point where you are suicidal, call Samaritans as it is easier to confide in a stranger sometimes. If you can talk to friends, that can be a support network.

Physically, smoking hash regularly will clog your lungs with tar, leading to lung disease. You may have a lowered immune response so constantly have colds, flu and infections. The chances of stroke and heart attacks increase from taking marijuana.

Studies show that if you try cannabis in your late teens or early twenties you are more likely to try other drugs, like cocaine later. It's not worth it.

Cocaine is sourced from the coca leaves of the South American plant Erythroxylon coca. Cocaine hydrochloride is a drug that's become fashionable or cool to snort in towns and cities across Europe. People in high powered jobs with unlimited cash and deadlines tend to take it the same way some of us have a glass of wine to relax. It can make you feel articulate, buzzy and invincible, but it's short lived.

Amazingly, it was used as an ingredient in the initial form of coca cola. By the way, coca cola is a fabulous cleaner for metal as it strips years of grime and dirt within minutes. Zero Coca cola is one of the poisons of our time. Clever marketing and advertising manipulate you into thinking it's cool. It's not. Read the chapter on SUGAR which is also addictive and a poison.

You might think it fun to snort a line of coke at a party after a few drinks. If you do, you could later face a situation over which you have little control. Cocaine is addictive. It's a fine, white powder also known as snow, powder, coke or blow. If you experiment with it in your late teens you're more likely to become hooked, addicted, and to try other drugs.

Taking coke and alcohol together can be a lethal combination. If you're stupid enough to try it a few times, the mesolimbic dopamine system, which is the reward centre in your BRAIN, will change. The more you snort it, the more you'll need to function and to feel 'normal' or to get the 'high' you had the time before. If you try to give it up, the periods in between can turn you into a reclusive, angry, negative person. Snorting cocaine will become a gnawing need and focal point in your life, over riding the need to eat healthy food and to engage in authentic relationships with people.

As you take cocaine more often you'll experience isolation, where you lose touch with people and reality. Stress will worsen the addiction. Intense feelings of paranoia, irritability, panic attacks and mental health issues will be heightened.

On a physical level, snorting cocaine will interfere with your sense of smell, irritating your throat and nasal area, making swallowing awkward and causing nosebleeds. After a snort you might feel euphoric and alert but it's short lived. On a more serious level, people who use cocaine are more likely to have tremors, strokes, extreme chest and abdominal pain and heart attacks. You can die young from messing about with cocaine.

If you're studying at college or university or have a demanding, challenging job, cocaine will adversely affect your BRAIN. Retaining information and concentrating will become challenging. Your orbitofrontal cortex in the brain will be affected. You'll deny that there is a problem. Cocaine usage will cause neuroadaptations in neurons in your brain that release glutamate, which links to your reward system. Once addicted, you'll find it almost impossible to give up. DEBT could increase and your relationships and good health will decline. Think twice.

Most of us will take pharmaceutical pain killers every now again for menstrual cramps or headaches. I take paracetamol sometimes if I am desperate, but try to avoid it as it takes the liver, our main sorting and clearing house in the body, many hours to clear just one tablet. When we take a painkiller our opioid receptors are activated. Daily MEDITATION can be as effective for long term pain relief. I've spoken to people in the past who were given Valium for anxiety and were addicted to it for years. Check to see if anything you've been prescribed has side effects or is addictive. Pain killers containing codeine are addictive. Some medications contain diphenhydramine which is a chemical found in pharmaceutical products to alleviate the symptoms of colds and allergies and help you sleep. This should not be used in excess. Try to use HERBAL remedies and ESSENTIAL OILS instead.

There are many powerful, incredible pharmaceutical drugs that maintain and save lives. Some of these drugs have caused controversy due to the extortionate price of them. If you can, opt for more natural ALTERNATIVES for pain.

Antidepressants or selective serotonin reuptake inhibitors (SSRIs) change the serotonin levels in your BRAIN. An SSRI prevents the neurotransmitters serotonin, dopamine and norepinephrinefrom being naturally reabsorbed back into nerve cells. The neurotransmitter will stay in the synapse, the gap between the nerves. These are not addictive the way marijuana and cocaine are. Taking SSRIs may change the way you experience emotions. Your doctor may advise you to take them for three to six months. Use EXERCISE, MEDITATION and MINDFULNESS, a new hobby and a healthy diet with supplements of OMEGAS to maintain mental health.

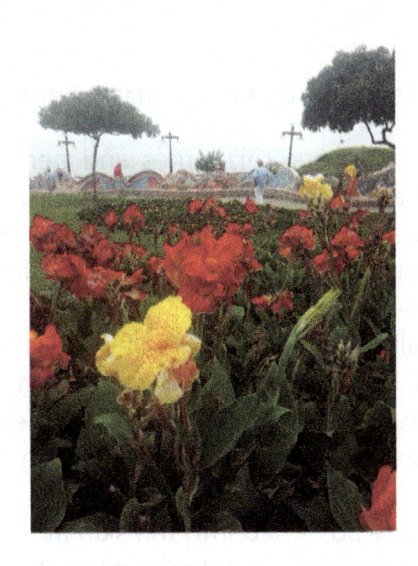

ESSENTIAL OILS

Scientists from the Federal University of Rio de Janeiro recently discovered that women have nearly 50% more brain cells in the part of their brain that processes aromas and smells than men do.

Essential oils have been used for spiritual, religious and healing medicinal purposes for thousands of years in cultures in ancient Egypt, India, Arabia and China. They were considered valuable in trade and exported and imported. Different oils were sourced in various parts of the world. The results of their uses have been passed down through empirical knowledge by herbalists and Arabic and medieval physicians. About 460 BC Hippocrates the "father of medicine" was said to have used these essences to heal. The Romans luxuriated in their scented baths and utilised many unguents, applying them to battle wounds.

Essential oils are the heart or essence of a plant; taken from the rind of the fruit, bark, twigs or leaves from trees, the petals of flowers, rhizomes and berries. Through the ages, man has perfected the art of aromatherapy and has developed the technical expertise so that these essences can be effectively extracted, distilled, blended and preserved.

Chemically, the components of the oils are powerful and should be used with respect and in the correct amounts, usually diluted in a base or carrier oil such as avocado, sweet almond, jojoba, wheat germ, grape seed or the HERB St. John's Wort.

The oils are absorbed into the skin at different rates but the capillaries will have drawn most of them into the system through the skin within 20 minutes to an hour. 70% of what we put onto our skin is absorbed into our bodies. If inhaled through the nose, the lungs will access the oils much faster. The oils are used in perfumes. Some oils are a "top" note which means they are volatile and will evaporate quickly forming your first 'impression', whilst others are "middle" notes, the heart, and finally the "base" notes which fix a perfume. It's these which give the lingering scent of the perfume hours after it has been applied.

"The roof of the internal nose is lined with a thin layer of mucous. Into this mucous project very tiny hairs. It is not certain whether the hairs project beyond the mucous, or simply into it. They form the tip of the rod like olfactory nerve cells, and there are between six and twelve hairs to each cell. The hairs are unprotected extensions of the actual neural cells, so that olfaction is exceptional among the senses in that it involves an extremely direct interaction between the neuron and the source of stimulation. The other end of each neuron leads directly to the olfactory bulb in the brain. Olfactory stimulation, then, has the capacity to produce immediate and direct effect on the nervous system."

"The Art of Aromatherapy" by Robert Tisserand*

The chemical components of the essence will then interact with the body's chemistry and affect and benefit certain organs and systems. The oils therefore are beneficial pharmacologically, physiologically and psychologically. I have always enjoyed using the oils in my daily routines whether it's in the bath, in a burner or on my wrists as a perfume. Always dilute them on the skin and put plenty of water in your burner and keep it topped up. I also use them in facial creams and products, adding a drop or two to what I already have, as they are potent. They vary in price in relation to how cheap the source is and how much of the original material is needed to make a certain amount. For instance, rose is more expensive than lemon due to the contrast in the price of the fruit and flowers and the amount of petals needed. If I have a cold, viral infection or sinusitis I put the oils in a bowl of boiled water and sit with my head under a towel over the steam, which works as an expectorant and is very effective and beneficial. Tisserand have a wide range of quality oils and most health food shops sell ranges in 5 ml or 10 ml bottles. Check to see if they are undiluted as some of the more expensive oils are sold diluted. Most oils are sold in their undiluted form so invest in a variety of base or carrier oils. A safe guide to use is 10 drops of essential oil in 20 ml of base oil. Only use the oils with the guidance of a therapist if pregnant.

Below are listed the primary oils that I've used over the years as an ITEC Aromatherapist and personally, for a variety of uses. I've included the Latin names as there are different varieties and types of plants.

BASIL, French. Ocimum basilicum

This refreshing, uplifting herb is also known as sweet basil and in India is used in Ayurvedic practise as Tulsi. It's perhaps one of the best oils for the nervous system providing support, clarity and healing on a mental, emotional level as it is fortifying and strengthening. I use it as a "pick me up" and also as an effective oil to clear headaches, lungs and sinuses. Basil is beneficial for asthma, coughs and bronchitis due to its affinity with the respiratory system. It's also an antidepressant, helpful for mental fatigue and useful for fevers, nausea, vomiting and earache. This oil has a strong scent and I only use a drop or two in burners, as a steam inhalation for colds and flu and in the bath. I like to blend it with eucalyptus and lavender.

BERGAMOT. Citrus bergamia

This oil is taken from the rind of the fruit and has a light, floral, citrusy aroma. It's an extremely useful oil with a beautiful scent and is effective against SKIN, mouth, respiratory and URINARY tract infections. In a blend with juniper and lavender I've used it for psoriasis and eczema and mixed it with tea tree and chamomile for acne. It's beneficial for sore throats and tonsillitis. I put a few drops in a teaspoonful of avocado oil on my neck and throat and use it as a gargle in a teaspoon of colloidal silver or coconut oil as a mouthwash. As a nerve sedative it's valuable for depression and anxiety so I use it in my bath with clary sage and geranium, which smells divine. This is an important oil for women as it can be helpful for thrush, cystitis, leucorrhoea (discharge) and vaginal irritation. Avoid putting it on your skin if you're on the beach and sunbathing, as it can increase the photosensitivity of the skin.

CHAMOMILE, ROMAN.
Chamaemelum nobile

This oil was used by the Egyptians and Moors and was one of the nine sacred herbs for the Saxons. This ancient plant is indicated for heavy, painful periods or scanty, irregular flow as it balances excess. It's beneficial during MENOPAUSE. If I'm feeling nervous, agitated, irritated and unable to SLEEP I blend this soothing, calming oil with lavender and smooth it onto my face, chest and abdomen. It's a superb oil for headaches, inflammation, chilblains, dermatitis and reddened, sensitive skin. If you're stressed put a few drops in a warm bath at night. Chamomile is helpful for neuralgia (pain along nerves) arthritis, joint and muscular pain. I blend it with ginger for sprains after applying an icepack. Mixed with Bergamot and Fennel it can be used for dyspepsia, colic and indigestion. This oil is linked to the spleen and liver and is said to be helpful in engorgement of the liver and jaundice.

CLARY SAGE Salvia Sclarea

One of my favourite oils for women with a warm, nutty aroma, Clary sage is a 'euphoric' so excellent for convalescence, menopause, PMS, depression, stress and anxiety. Use it for scanty or painful periods and during labour to soothe and initiate the birth. Avoid it if you're pregnant or recovering from cancer where oestrogen is a factor. Helpful for sore throats and asthma so put it in a burner. It's also best to avoid ALCOHOL if using this oil. Otherwise, this is a wonderful addition to your bath oil, as it's soothing and comforting.

CYPRESS Cupressus sempervirens

This oil is also beneficial for menstrual and menopausal problems, nervous tension and unequalled in its use for the treatment of varicose veins and haemorrhoids, due to its styptic nature and stimulation of the lymphatic and circulatory systems. Cypress is the best oil when there's been an excessive loss of fluid whether menstrual flow, bleeding, diarrhoea or perspiration. It has an affinity with the URINARY system, a sedative effect and smells similar to pine but is more pleasant. It is also refreshing in the bath with Eucalyptus and Basil if you have a cough, cold or chest infection. If a client has red thread veins and congestion in capilliaries or acne rosacea, I blend this oil with lavender, geranium and chamomile (German) in aloe vera and carrot oil for them. Cypress was highly prized in ancient civilizations and is still used by Tibetans in purification incense.

EUCALYPTUS, BLUE GUM Eucalyptus Globulus var.globulus

A household remedy in Australia, it's one of the most potent oils for bacterial and viral infections and for catarrh, coughs, asthma, throat infections and bronchitis as it's an excellent decongestant. Sprayed in the air or in a burner it will clear the bacteria staphylococci from an area. Use it in the bath for aching muscles, rheumatoid arthritis and poor circulation. On the skin this powerful oil helps heal herpes, chicken pox, burns, blisters and insect bites, as it's also cooling and refreshing. It can be used as an insect repellent, clears pustular conditions and is helpful when there's a fever. Combined with Bergamot, Tea Tree and Juniper in a bath it's effective in clearing genito-urinary infections. I've had amazing results with painful neuralgia and toothache after blending this oil with Chamomile and Clove and applying it to my face twice daily for a week.

GERANIUM Pelargonium graveolens

This is a really useful and beautiful green, floral aromatic oil for women and it is helpful for anxiety, MENOPAUSE, PMT, menorrhagia, (excessive blood loss during menstruation), engorgement of BREASTS and oedema (fluid retention). It contains the flavenoid Quercetin which is anti-inflammatory. Apply it to bruises along with Marjoram and with Cypress for broken capillaries and haemorrhoids. If you have been suffering from "burn out" or worn out adrenal function from over loading yourself, blend Geranium with Clary sage and a drop of Ginger in a warm bath every day. This oil is excellent for the SKIN for cold sores, shingles, acne, dermatitis, eczema, ulcers and wounds. I have used it for Candida. I blend it with Frankincense and Myrrh for a night moisturiser in sweet almond oil. Look for the Bourbon oil when purchasing Geranium as it's considered superior.

GINGER Zingiber officinale

After I've iced a sprain or injury I gently apply 5 drops of ginger in a teaspoon of sweet almond oil and then apply a bandage to hold the area in place. This is an outstanding oil for sprains, strain, arthritis, rheumatism, muscular aches and poor circulation. It's a hot, healing oil which is also effective in balancing the digestive system, so I use it as a belly rub or a few drops in the bath for diarrhoea, colic, flatulence, nausea, indigestion, travel and morning sickness. Ginger is refreshing and re-energising, so use it for physical and mental fatigue and exhaustion. A beneficial oil for colds, chills, catarrh, sinusitis and sore throats, it's an expectorant and stimulant.

FENNEL Foeniculum vulgare

I've included fennel as it is an ancient herb and seed oil, although we now just use the sweet oil, not the bitter variety. It has an affinity with the liver, spleen and gall bladder and has been used for anorexia and constipation. It stimulates the appetite and either relieves spasms in the digestive area or improves peristalsis, the movement of the intestines to ensure complete elimination. If you suffer from constipation, drink psyillium husks mixed with a litre of water and use Fennel in a base oil to massage from the right side of the belly to the top left, down to the left hip then across the lower abdomen to the right hip. Use firm sweeping strokes. If you are on a weight loss plan and feel bloated and have a problem with cellulite, blend this oil with Cypress and Juniper for your baths. Fennel is also known as a galactogogue which means it has an oestrogenic effect improving the flow of a nursing mother's milk. If you're concerned about oestrogenically linked cancer it's advisable to avoid Fennel, Clary sage and Geranium for awhile. Otherwise it's another oil to include if you're traversing the menopause and looking for ALTERNATIVES to HRT.

FRANKINCENSE Boswellia carteri

One of the most effective anti- ageing and rejuvenating oils for skin care, this oil is extracted from the gum or resin of a tree. It was a highly valued oil in ancient times and was in use 5,000 years ago. I use it for dry, mature skin in masks and moisturizers blending it with myrrh and avocado oil for wrinkles and tired skin. Also helpful for healing ulcers and wounds it was used in ancient times for its regenerative properties. In a spiritual context it deepens the breath, so is conducive to meditation and prayer. Soothing for stress, tension and anxiety, it's a warm, dry oil so beneficial for asthma, bronchitis, catarrh, coughs and laryngitis as well as assisting in clearing IRINARY infections and STDs such as Gonorrhoea. It has similar properties to myrrh.

LAVENDER Lavender angustifolia

The word Lavender comes from the Latin "lavare" which means to wash. The Romans used this oil in their elaborate bathing sessions and may have introduced it to Britain but France is now the main producer. I have found it one of the best oils to comfort and sooth agitation, hysteria and for insomnia and irritability. It's also helpful for nervous tension, headaches and migraines, earache and epilepsy. Studies showed that if lavender could be associated with calm by using it linked to massage and relaxation techniques, epileptics could use it when they anticipated an attack. This proved effective in reducing episodes. Lavender is probably one of the most versatile essential oils as it is antiseptic, mildly analgesic and an antidepressant. It can be used on all manner of skin conditions to rebalance and calm but is particularly good for reddened, sensitive skin when blended with Chamomile (German). As it's a decent cytophylactic (regenerates skin cells), it's useful in homemade moisturisers and skin care and unparalleled for healing burns. Never put any kind of vegetable oil on a burn but run cool water over it first and apply lavender in Aloe Vera, if some is to hand, after a few minutes. Apply a drop of Lavender to sooth insect bites and stings and in the bath for sunburn. This oil benefits all the systems through the body by restabilising, as it's an adaptogen, maintaining balance. If you have VAGINAL leucorrhoea (discharge) use it in your bath with Bergamot.

MARJORAM Origanum marjoram

This is an excellent oil for bruises, sprains, stiff joints and aching muscles. It can be helpful for the digestion, lessening heartburn or indigestion and flatulence. Avoid it during pregnancy. I have used it in blends for massage for arthritis and rheumatism. Added to a drop of thyme, which can be harsh, it is also comforting and alleviates chesty coughs and bronchitis. If you're not sleeping and feel stressed and tense, blend it with a couple of drops of lavender. This is also an effective combination for headaches. Marjoram is also helpful for torticollis, a condition where the neck muscles tighten.

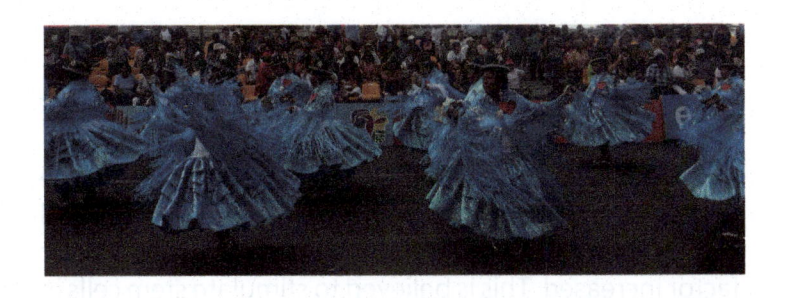

EXERCISE

Walking briskly a few times a week for twenty to forty minutes has many benefits. Not only does it lift your mood and alleviate depression, a common problem in our times of high expectations, consumerism and lack of connectedness in communities, it has proven physical benefits. It's cheap, and if you can do it outside of a city, you get fresh air and sunshine. Make sure you get some sun on your skin to get the health enhancing effects of Vitamin D. Sun block should obviously be used if you're sat on a beach for eight hours but let the sun warm your skin for twenty minutes without it first. Sunscreen can be CHEMICAL laden too, so find a good quality one.

A study on regular walkers showed that the hippocampus, which is a part of the BRAIN used for memory, expanded. MRI scans actually showed that the brains of regular walkers looked younger than those of couch potatoes and people who never exercised. In another study with MRI scans, tests highlighted that mental stress and anxiety shrink the brain!

In studies and research on FASTING, where you have only five hundred calories in a twenty four hour period twice a week, the protein, brain derived neurotrophic factor increased. This is believed to stimulate stem cells in the hippocampus. Could fasting and exercise combined help prevent dementia, senility and Alzheimers? Many people believe so after years of studies. Brain derived neurotrophic factor seems to protect the brain and improves mood and lowers anxiety.

Walk barefoot on the earth, grass and sand whenever you can as it's now believed to be beneficial as free electrons and energy are drawn up from the earth to rejuvenate you. Bare foot running is becoming more popular but research it before you try it.

We have three different types of muscle fibres; slow, fast and superfast. The superfast muscle fibres are white and are used when you perform short burst exercises. The latest research shows that interval training and exercising in short bursts for around thirty seconds (where your heart rate increases to your anaerobic threshold, so that you're breathless), followed by a slower pace of ninety seconds is more beneficial for fat burning and health. High intensity interval training boosts human growth hormone for optimal health. Doing this eight times in your exercise session, whether you're running, dancing or on a bike, is more effective for maintaining weight loss results than walking sedately for an hour or two.

There is also a type of fat known as brown fat. Brown fat cells are full of mitochondria, the engines in our cells so this type of fat burns energy and produces heat so burning calories. People with lower body mass indexes

EXERCISE

(BMI) have more brown fat. You could increase the efficiency of your brown fat by keeping the temperature cool where you live and exercising in cold weather. In animal studies exercise converted white fat cells to brown.

My version of interval training entails running as fast as I can for the thirty seconds, then walking for ninety seconds and repeating this seven times as am incapable of long distance running. I have always included weight training in my life as it's one of the best things you can do to prevent OSTEOPOROSIS or brittle bones and breakages later in life.

I've had ME or chronic fatigue syndrome for thirty years so exercising is not always an option. It's important to recognise signs when you have ME. If you start to feel fatigued it can be challenging just to walk up a flight of stairs or maintain a coherent conversation. Go to bed for a couple of hours if you have ME, so that you recover before exercising again. Regular exercise does help lift your mood and stimulate endorphins.

Muscle weighs more than fat and weight training continues to burn calories even after you've finished your session. You will become more toned by weight training and your main focus should be on how well your clothes fit and not necessarily what the scales say. Some advocate exercising on an empty stomach, as ultimately your goal is to re-educate your body to burn both fat and sugar. If you drink coffee, having a black one without food may increase fat burning. Eating prior to exercise will mean that your body will focus on burning off any of the sugar content rather than building muscle.

Many of us are insulin and leptin resistant. These two are important HORMONES. Exercise helps to stabilise insulin levels. Start with light weights after taking advice from a trainer (or learning online) and gradually build up your repetitions. If you just want strength not bulk, do three sets of twelve repetitions with a lighter weight. Squats and lunges target the buttocks and legs and abdominal crunches are important for your 'core'. Simply lie on your back with your legs bent, feet on the ground and hands on the side thighs and slowly lift your head and shoulders up off the floor and build up your repetitions. Ask your trainer to show you 'the plank'.

You may well find that any painful back issues are lessened when you strengthen your core. Most women need to target the back of the arms more to tone the triceps. Vary your program so you work on different areas and muscle groups and try it two or three times a week, interspersed with some brisk walking, circuit training or interval training. Ask a trainer or Pilate's teacher to show you a routine 'on the ball' to target muscles and core for variety. Vibrational plate machines offer an effective alternative to weight training in studios.

Avoid fruit and sugar before and after your workout but ensure you drink enough WATER after your workout. Include a weekly YOGA or Pilate's session to elongate muscles and to maintain core strength. At the very least take the stairs at work or walk the dog daily.

FASTING

There have been a number of long term studies and a lot of research on the controversial subject of fasting and reducing your calories. I was sceptical initially, being a "grazer" and eating five small meals a day and if low, premenstrual and moody, large portions of cake, ice-cream and chocolate. Many of my friends were losing weight and bounding around energised after starting the 5:2 program and new way of eating. They were elated that they could maintain their ideal weight with a relatively small amount of will power and self discipline. Other people seem to benefit from eating five small meals spread out over the day. Experiment with both options and keep a FOOD DIARY.

The research indicates that fasting is beneficial not just for weight loss to get into the pair of jeans you bought five years ago, but in anti- ageing and prevention and alleviation of chronic, debilitating and degenerative diseases. If you follow this plan you still eat exactly what you like on your five non fast days and consume five hundred calories in twenty four hours on two non consecutive days. This is known to mildly stress the body.

When you fast, "repair" genes and responses in the body will be activated, so that regeneration can take place. We have around one hundred million million cells in our bodies and they are miniscule worlds in themselves. There are two hundred different kinds of cells and they busy themselves with taking in nutrients and protecting us from pathogens that might enter our blood stream. Our bodies, tissues and bones are being constantly replaced as these cells self destruct and rebuild, which is why we are what we eat. Cells are continually dividing and your Telomeres on your chromosomes which contain your DNA, will gradually shorten as you age.

Autophagy is the term used to describe this cleaning up and incredible constant maintenance that takes place every second as a cell will either self destruct or remove a damaged part to renew. When cells multiply and this process fails it can cause "overgrowth" or tumours which can either be cancerous and malignant, or benign, and so just taking up space. In a relatively short space of time and with little effort we could reduce our chances of suffering diabetes, heart disease, Alzheimer's and cancer by fasting, upping our vegetable intake and taking moderate, regular EXERCISE. We could live longer, more productive, energetic lives.

When you fast for twelve to fourteen hours IGF-1(a hormone in your body) levels drop and the body goes into repair mode. IGF-1 or insulin like growth factor may be linked to the development of disease. The hormone that's produced during fasting FG21 could be the link to a longer life but research is ongoing. Fibroblast growth factor increases when you are cold and is thought to improve insulin sensitivity and glucose intolerance. Brown fat may become more efficient at burning calories when you spend time in a cold environment. Being a bit chilly also increases a substance in our systems known

FASTING

as irisin which builds lean muscle, converts white fat to brown and enhances bone density.

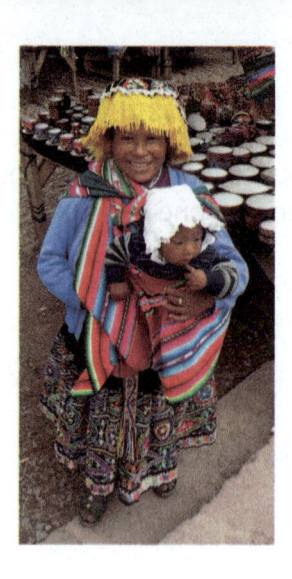

FERTILITY

Women are delaying that period in their lives when they think about conceiving and starting a family because many of them have successful, well paid jobs. Women have a huge amount to contribute to more senior management jobs and the amount working in well paid, powerful positions in businesses and politics is on the increase. The discrepancy in pay still needs to be addressed as women doing the same job as men are sometimes paid 20% less. You may have made the decision not to have children early in life, due to a passion for a path or chosen career.

After the age of thirty your chances of conceiving naturally will start to drop and by forty, the chances are lower. If you haven't met The Man by then, you may have to accept that you won't have children and you purposely create a fulfilling life with friends, travel, spending time on things you enjoy and which inspire and stimulate you. You may reach the age of forty five and feel regret that

FERTILITY

you didn't conceive, but we all have a choice regarding how and what we think, and acceptance, and making the best of our lives exactly as they are, is the only option unless you're willing to adopt or pay for IVF.

If you are planning a baby it's an exciting time and the beginning of an adventure. Discussions with your partner are essential, so that you both know your expectations of each other as a rough template and you expect that your relationship may be put 'on hold' somewhat due to lack of sleep and new responsibilities. Patience and support are important so that you each feel involved to the point that you need and want to be. If you are expecting your partner to change nappies, run the bath routine with the rubber duck and stay in once a week so you have a night off, state it clearly and listen to what his expectations and hopes are too.

If you need to lose weight before conceiving, that will be your first priority and a doctor will advise you on this. Start an exercise plan with a friend to motivate you and make it fun. You can work out the window of time in which you are ovulating by counting fourteen days from the start of your period.

Take a good multi vitamin and mineral and increase folic acid as a supplement. Lack of folate has been linked to birth defects. Folate may help protect the foetus against neural tubular defect where the two sides of the body fuse leading to spina bifida. Folic acid may be included in your multi vitamin and mineral, but you can take up to 400 ug a day whilst trying to conceive and then up to the twelfth week in the pregnancy. To increase Folate in your diet, eat more asparagus, broccoli, cauliflower and Brussels sprouts.

The MINERAL Selenium plays a key role in fertility, as it increases sperm quality and sperm count, so give your man Brazil nuts and cashews to snack on and ask him to take a Selenium and VITAMIN D supplement, along with his multi VITAMIN and mineral supplement.

New studies show that taking OMEGA 3 during pregnancy could offset childhood obesity.

If you've been trying for a while and are feeling frustrated, book a reflexology treatment once a month to boost your chances, to enhance your health generally and to relax you. Make an appointment with an acupuncturist too, to discuss this route. Some people reduce coffee, drugs, cigarettes and alcohol after they get the good news that they are pregnant, as these may be implicated in early miscarriage or birth defects in your child.

Wash vegetables in vinegar and lemon juice then rinse well or buy mainly organic to reduce your intake of herbicides and pesticides, as they act as oestrogen mimics, which may have contributed to unbalancing your reproductive system. Phytosterols in VEGETABLES help prevent reproductive damage from these toxins.

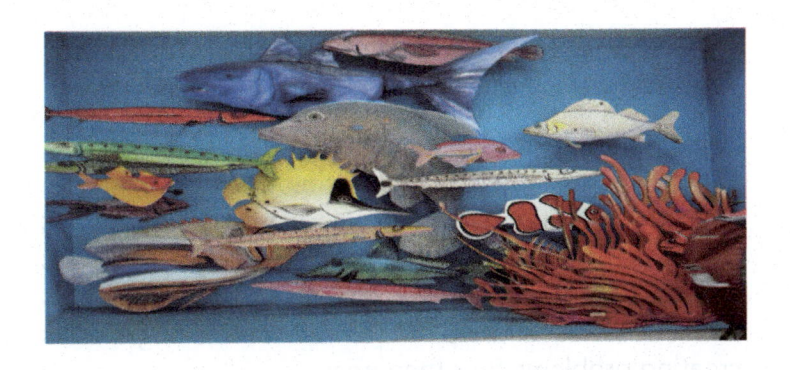

FISH

Mercury has been found in Tuna, Swordfish and Barracuda in amounts which are not acceptable for regular human consumption. Cod has been over fished. There is also a concern about anchovies and herring being depleted to feed farmed tuna and salmon. One third of fishing stocks has collapsed. The price of fish makes it difficult for families on a tight budget to enjoy it every week. Unless you eat wild Alaskan sockeye salmon, most of the fish you buy will be from a fish farm unless stated otherwise. This is now big business as the global demand increases. Farmed fish may have been fed soy, corn or produce with low levels of OMEGA 3.

Wild fish get their Omega 3 from aquatic plants. Many people are deficient in Omega 3 which is key to optimal mental and physical health. It's now thought that childhood obesity may be linked to the mother having insufficient levels of Omega 3 during pregnancy. We already have enough Omega 6 in our general diet, but farmed fish can accumulate levels of the wrong fatty acids in their tissue, creating an unbalanced diet for us.

Farmed fish are also fed antibiotics as they live in crowded conditions in their own waste products. This could lead to antibiotic-resistant disease in us. This is also a problem in the meat industry. These antibiotics and chemicals end up in the sea and along coasts creating problems for other areas.

It will also mean that farmed fish may harbour disease which may be transferred to the natural population of sea life. Limit fish to once or twice a week, buy freshly caught fish as a treat if possible, and get creative with vegetables.

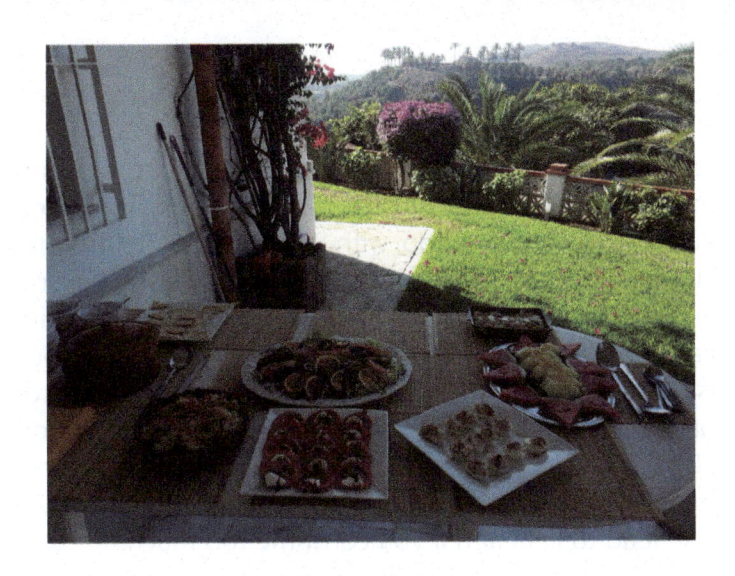

FOOD

The Glycaemic index (GI) is a way of calculating the rate at which carbohydrates are digested and converted into SUGAR by your body. Low GI foods have little or no sugar so insulin from the pancreas is stable. These include lean white poultry, fish, eggs, seeds, NUTS, VEGETABLES, berries and dark CHOCOLATE.

Cereals such as oats, wheat, rye and barley have a medium level GI. Have days where you omit these. When carbohydrates are eaten, they turn into SUGAR. The excess SUGAR makes your pancreas works overtime. Excess sugar and carbohydrates in your diet turn into layers of fat on your body and increase your risk of dealing with diabetes as you become insulin resistant. Avoid fruit juices, corn syrup, maltose, boxed cereals and fried foods. Start to check and research the long list of ADDITIVES on the back of packets.

You need a gradual release of energy so choose brown rice instead of white, have quinoa in soups and salads and avoid eating cakes, biscuits, puddings and milk chocolate every day. Quinoa is a high fibre seed and is high in protein too, with 8 grams of protein in one cup and is an alternative to bulk meals out, as it's filling and nutritious. Buck wheat is another alternative to white carbohydrates with 6 grams of protein per cup. Humous is a healthy snack in small amounts and has 7 grams of protein in two tablespoons. Lentils and beans are good alternatives to red meat. Lentils have around 18 grams of protein per cup. Don't overdo eating protein as it can also lead to ill health if you consume too much.

The body cannot make nine of the twenty amino acids that make up protein, so we need to get them from our diet, in various forms through the week. Eat Tempeh, which is fermented soya and has thirty one grams of protein per cup, in stews. Only use NON genetically modified soya. These two are excellent healthy alternatives to eggs and meat. Snack on Chia seeds which have 2 grams of protein in a tablespoon or add them to porridge with a small handful of chopped Brazil nuts, walnuts, almonds and macadamia NUTS.

If you eliminate wheat from your diet for a month, then reintroduce it, and have intolerance problems, it may be time to cut it from your diet. Notice if you have bloating after reintroducing it. Wheat in any form will cause your blood sugar levels to shoot up which is also linked to ill health as it causes "spikes" in Insulin.

If you're on a mission to lose weight or trying hard to maintain weight loss, try having two hard boiled or poached eggs for breakfast, giving you more energy as it is protein. It's a fallacy that you have to avoid fat if you want to lose weight. Include a small handful of mixed NUTS a few times a week. Eat a small amount of full fat, good quality cheese in a salad with avocados. These are satisfying, healthy fats. I include hard goat's cheese in salads and add it to tomato dishes. It's easy to grow tomatoes in large pots and bags. Try growing your own vegetables.

Garcinia cambogia is a fruit containing Hydroxycitric acid (HCA). It can aid in weight loss, so if you are obese or need to lose belly fat to maintain health, it could be useful. It blocks the enzyme citrate lyase, which turns starches and SUGAR into fat. It may increase levels of serotonin the contentment neurotransmitter and mildly suppress appetite.

Serotonin lowers food cravings. Take 1.5 grams of garcinia cambogia three times a day on an empty stomach. Take it half an hour before you eat and look for a supplement with potassium and magnesium with low lactone. Ensure you're taking a quality multi VITAMIN and MINERAL supplement too.

Ditch fat free commercial products as these can contain sweeteners which are actually toxic to your system. Avoid commercial cereals with added sugars and just eat small amounts of jumbo oats. Oats are a good source of the B VITAMINS which help to keep you calm but focussed. They also contain Inositol which metabolises fat and reduces your chances of heart disease. We need the MINERALS Phosphorus, Calcium and Iron. Read the chapter on XYLITOL for alternatives to SUGAR.

Have a small amount of porridge oats an hour before bed, with full fat milk or almond or COCONUT milk, as the carbohydrates have a relaxing effect on your system. I soak my few tablespoons of uncooked jumbo oats in berry tea overnight and the following day add a handful of blueberries or raspberries, a sprinkle of flax seed, pumpkin or sunflower seeds and a small handful of mixed NUTS that I've soaked in water. This makes the nuts easier to digest. Add a blob of natural yogurt. This version of burcher muesli has all the ingredients for a tasty, healthy snack which I can have late afternoon.

Don't buy commercial yogurt with added fruit as these can contain high levels of sugar and high fructose corn syrup. Avoid low fat yogurt and foods as these normally contain sweeteners, which you need to eliminate from your diet. You need to avoid these by checking the labels on food. I eat natural, plain yogurt with whole fruit as a sweet afternoon snack, on days when I find it tough not to eat a large bar of dark chocolate instead of just a square. If possible, it's best to eat whole fruit on an empty stomach, not after a large meal, as fruit passes through your stomach within half an hour.

There is a link between your mental and emotional state and food. Binge eating can occur if you feel hopeless and helpless in situations where you feel you have no control. This can lead to weight gain. Keep a DIARY of how you feel and the exact amounts of what, and when you eat, to verify this. MINDFULNESS is really important here to recognise triggers that make you reach for comfort or junk food. Ask yourself if you'll enjoy it and how you'll feel afterwards.

If you're aiming to lose weight it can be helpful to keep a photo of when you were at your ideal weight on the fridge door or to keep an item of clothing you want to wear again hanging in view in the bedroom when you feel tempted. Body image and acceptance of things we can't change need to be addressed. Advertising in magazines frequently show AIRBRUSHED and enhanced

FOOD

pictures of women leading to poor self image in average women. If you have a daughter, keep an eye on her eating habits and attitude to food so you can help her avoid the extremes of either obesity or anorexia, bulimia and unhelpful yo yo or fad dieting.

There are a number of super foods you can easily include in your weekly diet. Tumeric contains an incredible compound, curcumin. You can add this to black pepper, COCONUT oil or milk and in soups, stews or curries. The spice turmeric boosts your immune system to fight infection and is a natural painkiller. It reduces inflammation thought to contribute to disease, aids healthy digestion, joint mobility, fights cancer and detoxifies the liver. It also regulates metabolism and keeps cholesterol levels stable. Tumeric may enhance brain function and is a powerful ANTIOXIDANT.

GARLIC

This super food should be included in your weekly diet. Perhaps not recommended before a date, but otherwise soak up the beneficial manganese, calcium, phosphorus, selenium and VITAMINS B6 and C. Garlic contains Allicin which is a natural antibiotic and impressive anti oxidant. It battles infection from viruses, bacteria and fungus and helps prevent cancers of the pancreas, BRAIN, BREAST and lungs.

Many people these days have mineral deficiencies and seem to have a constant runny, red nose, colds and flu. Garlic is also good for your thyroid gland which regulates metabolism.

Keep a beady eye on your bones as you head into your late forties and to avoid OSTEOPOROSIS, eat garlic and take a supplement with the MINERALS, calcium, magnesium, boron and vitamin D. You also need to include weight bearing exercise to avoid osteoporosis because you can't play badminton or go on a date with a broken hip.

Inflammation in your body is linked to disease and garlic reduces it, boosts your immune system, improves cardiovascular health and reduces blood pressure. It's tasty too so include it in your soups, stews and curries but don't overcook it. Garlic helps to cleanse the blood and remove Mercury and Lead from your system which are detrimental to the functioning and health of your kidneys, bowel and liver.

Aged black garlic from Korea may be easier to use as ideally you must crush the garlic to release the goodies, and then eat within the hour without overcooking it. Aged garlic contains more sulphur and is fermented and fermented food is something else you should include weekly. It acts as a chelator removing heavy metals from your system. In studies black garlic reduced tumours. It also contains alli cycteine and is well absorbed and assimilated by the body.

If you have a toxic, acidic system from eating meat, drinking cocktails in happy hour and living in a polluted city, garlic helps to alkalise your system as it may be acidic. Disease thrives in acidity. Simply eat more vegetables to increase alkalinity in your body and mix a teaspoon of bicarbonate of soda mixed with fresh lemon juice in water and drink it once a month.

GENETICALLY ENGINEERED

A great deal of the soya and corn in our food these days is genetically engineered and it's hard to know just how much it will affect our cells and long term health. The agricultural chemical Glyphosate may affect the beneficial gut and BOWEL bacteria which is essential to optimal health and our immune response. Soya and corn may contain this chemical if it is genetically engineered. Check labels for non genetically modified (non GMO) when you buy soya milk and soy products.

Oestrogens in unfermented soya can block the thyroid hormones and its function. Soya is sometimes recommended to menopausal women because it contains Isoflavones which are plant oestrogens. I tend to drink miso soup and eat tempeh now, as they are fermented products and very beneficial for optimal health. There are excellent soya supplements on the market for MENOPAUSAL women, just ensure that any soya you use is non Genetically engineered.

Hydrogenated soybean oil is a transfat and damaging to your system. Don't buy or fry this product.

Margarine has been advertised as a health food for years now as an alternative to butter, when in fact it's highly processed. Avoid it. Hydrogenated products interfere with enzymes that fight cancer. They cause inflammation, increase bad cholesterol and make any

GENETICALLY ENGINEERED

health promoting Omega 3 fats less effective. Use butter sparingly. We tend to have a lot of Omega 6 in our diets and soyabean oil is a prime example. What we actually need is more Omega 3. Cook with butter or COCONUT OIL and ditch anything else. Flax and hemp seed oils are the best to use for salad dressings and in smoothies. Hemp has a protein profile similar to human blood and contains all essential amino acids, two key globulins, albumin and edestin which can repair our DNA. Hemp also contains the ideal ratio of the OMEGA essential fatty acids and IRON, magnesium and ZINC.

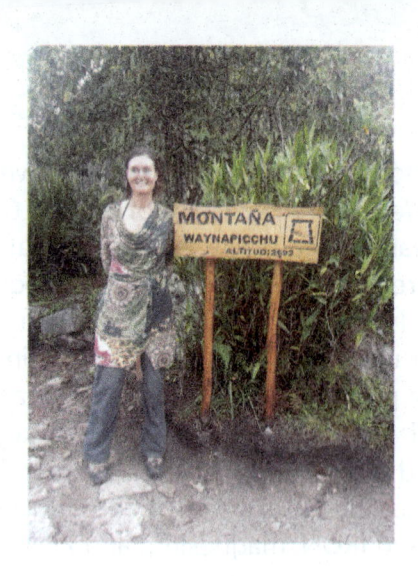

GOALS

What do you want in the next ten, twenty or thirty years? Have you thought about it recently? Some people drift through life unsure of that question and others have a calling to do a certain thing at a young age. Take a piece of paper and write a list of things you've thought of in the past and a list of things you love and enjoy. Travelling to Cambodia, learning how to play the guitar, getting a puppy and training it, running a marathon or learning a language? Goal setting and achievements can be markers through life, and will give you inspiration and satisfaction.

Self development ensures that you stay curious and attempt to be the best that you can be. Your goal might be to walk half an hour every day, join the local choir or crochet group or give up smoking. It doesn't matter what it is, goals can enhance your life by flexing your will power, cultivating focus and introducing you to people you'd never have met sat on the sofa in front of a soap

GOALS

opera. After you've made your list, take action and write the plan out with details and a time frame if needed.

Make a goal board with pictures and photos and notes so that you see it every day. Imagine the benefits and happiness linked to your goal then tell yourself it's done! Visualise in your mind, running across the finishing line or buying that dress, or how it will feel to trek in New Zealand or paint a watercolour.

To be content and grateful with what you have now is a kind of success. Perception of success varies from person to person. Set achievable goals but dare to dream big too.

We spend a large chunk of our time at work and it can impact all aspects of your health and well being. It's important to make time to do nothing too. In the next decade more and more people will work part time or have two different jobs, as they spend half their week on entrepreneurial projects. Try to volunteer in some way, sometime in your life. It's excellent life experience and can add to your curriculum vitae (CV).

If your goal is to get a fulfilling, interesting job you'll need to develop decent listening and communication skills. Most of us don't listen properly as we're thinking ahead to our answer, or contribution to a conversation.

Before you go to an interview, research the company and show awareness and some understanding of their ethics and goals. Be authentic and be yourself. Ask yourself how you could contribute and improve and enhance the company. Whilst in the interview, relax by staying aware of your breath so that you can smile occasionally. Be clear and concise with any questions and responses, demonstrating that you are listening and that you have initiative, but can also be an asset in a team.

If you're applying for a job in management the interviewer will need to see that you are calm, so you could work under pressure and to deadlines. You may be asked what you would do in an imaginary scenario. Problem sorting skills will be required, along with the ability to see situations from different angles. Knowing how to motivate and integrate people and to understand their skill sets and aptitudes will ensure you get optimal results for the individual in your team and the company. Being able to delegate, manage time and constantly lead by good example are management skills. People will remember you and connect with as a result of how you made them feel. Obviously, personal hygiene and appropriate clothing are essential.

A financial plan is prudent so whether it's a savings account, a jar under your bed stuffed with fivers or an ISA, stick with it. However old you are now, you can be sure that the system will change and the strain put on societies to look after their elderly and sick will be huge, so plan your nest egg, particularly if you're in your twenties and thirties. Don't make money your god. Money in itself is not evil and gives you freedom and the means to live comfortably, but if you're working twelve hours a day for ten years are you savouring life too? Work smart, not too hard, when you can.

Welcome abundance in whatever form it comes in and focus on what you'd like in a positive way, so you really believe in yourself and your ability to grow and learn and achieve. Be specific when goal setting and always imagine your THOUGHTS as physical things that can shape and mould your world for the better. The more

GOALS

you realise that you create what happens to you with your goals, positive thoughts, desires and intentions, the juicier your life will be, so take responsibility for it.

It's challenging to stay positive in today's world but keep going and don't give up, as some things take a while and you're just supposed to learn many things before you finally reach your goal. Sometimes, it's not those people who were top of the class academically that achieve, it's the people who just kept going after countless rejections and setbacks.

It doesn't matter how old you are, goal setting can rejuvenate your life. Failure is an intrinsic and inevitable part of life but prolonged and constant negativity will poison you, and make the people around begin to want to avoid you. Observe how often you whine and complain about things and whether you could change them or not.

Accept some failure in your life as a learning experience and ask yourself what you learnt from any upsetting situations. Remember, it's none of your business what other people think of you. Relax and "allow" whatever comes into your life as part of a greater plan for your higher good, even when it looks the opposite of your goals. If you can't change it, then embrace it and act as if you chose it for yourself. Change and death are the two things we can't avoid, so remember that every day, and moment, is precious.

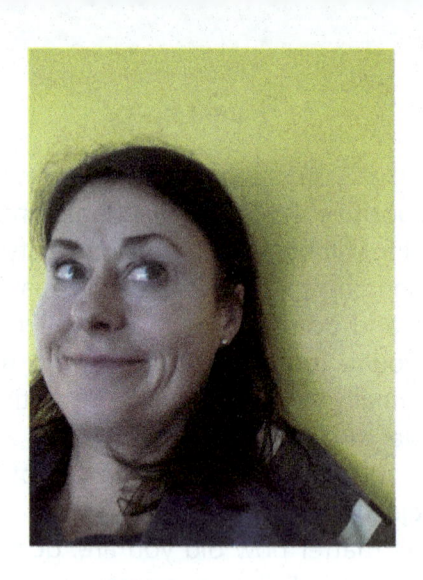

GRATITUDE

The dictionary defines gratitude as a "feeling of thankfulness or appreciation for gifts and favours". The latin root gratus means pleasing or thankful. In these times of instant self gratification, welfare benefits, children who demand designer trainers and capitalism, we seem to have forgotten how blessed we are. Some people realise from a young age that gratitude opens doors and allows them to accept that not everything will be handed to them on a plate.

Gratitude is a powerful practise and not just a new age term bandied around in a pseudo spiritual, sanctimonious way. We can affirm, notice and feel aware of gratitude every hour of every day. It will enhance your life and radiate outwards from you. Ben Stein said "Be grateful. Gratitude is the most powerful get rich scheme there is". To have a roof over our heads, clean water, enough food and emotional connections with other people and animals, is to live a rich life.

GRATITUDE

Watching the news recently may have triggered horrific awareness of refugees losing family, friends, limbs, homes and towns. Take time every day to feel thankful for all the positive things you have, and have had. Enjoy making future plans but feel grateful for how things are right now.

If you practise this and write in a DIARY regularly you'll naturally feel more contented, less depressed and happier. This will ripple out from you to those around you. Surround yourself with people who support and appreciate you and accept you for who you are. You can still feel grateful for those people who challenge or upset you, because all RELATIONSHIP is a mirror and an experience for you to learn and develop.

Before you begin your MEDITATION or MINDFULNESS practise take time to be thankful for the positive, uplifting people in your life and the small events and moments that enhance your experience of your day.

Keep a watchful "inner eye" on any thoughts that spiral around a victim mentality, a "poor me" attitude of doom and gloom. It takes focus and effort to notice these negative THOUGHTS and emotions and to keep replacing them with positivity and gratitude. Beware of crying and moaning to your friends over the years, as even they will start to see you as toxic, and may avoid you simply because it's draining to be around constant self pitying negativity. Friends are there to support and bolster and we will experience perhaps devastating events during our lifetimes, which they will be there for. Our BRAINS are plastic and capable of constantly changing and your THOUGHTS are like programming which affect your physical wellbeing.

Recent studies and research with groups of people has shown that people who are grateful SLEEP better, EXERCISE more, look after themselves, have lower blood pressure and are healthier.

Look for the good and find the funny in your daily life. Notice the positives in people you are in RELATIONSHIPS with, and new people you meet. Try to see the benefits in situations even if they appear outwardly negative. Keep forgiving and moving on.

You are the root of your own inner joy and contentment. Take responsibility for your own happiness so that it's not based purely on others and their actions, thoughts and feelings. Gratitude can transform your life into something extraordinary.

GREEN TEA

High quality green tea contains ANTI OXIDENTS from polyphenols and flavonoids. The catchins in flavonoids are powerful substances in the battle against disease. They slow down the ageing process while they inhibit the growth of blood vessels that feed cancer tumours. Due to green teas' artery opening and relaxing properties, it could also help to prevent strokes and heart attacks, as it lowers blood pressure and increases fat oxidation.

If you're on a fat loss programme, drink a few mugs a day. If you need to, use XYLITOL or a sugar alternative and squeeze a tiny amount of lemon juice or sugar free cranberry juice in it. Once a week I add a splash of apple cider vinegar which is cleansing for your system. Use honey sparingly if you are trying to lose weight because agave syrup and honey are still sugars, so can ultimately be stored as fat. Try luo han or other alternatives to SUGAR.

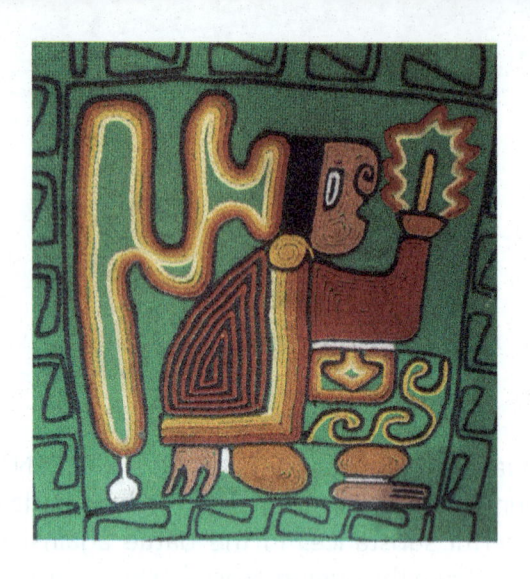

HERBS

Women have always used herbal remedies. The knowledge of them was empirical; passed down through generations to alleviate and heal a whole range of diseases and ailments. They were used in ancient rituals, can transform a meal and are still relevant as alternative medicine today. They have different actions and effects on mind and body. Some are calming, some stimulating and others antiseptic. Chinese medicine and western usage differs.

This is a concise, short list of herbs that link to the chapters in this book. I have included herbs so that if you are interested, you can research the subject further, along with homeopathics. Pharmaceutical DRUGS and painkillers are sometimes the only option, but herbs and ESSENTIAL OILS are natural plant chemicals, so can have a powerful effect.

There are reputable companies that have combined the correct amounts of these herbs in tinctures (liquid) or tablet supplements. Consult a homeopath or herbalist if you have decided to take this ALTERNATIVE, but very effective route.

Ashwagandha is used in Indian Ayurvedic medicine. In the ancient language Sanskrit, it translates from ashva which is horse and gandha, meaning smell. I take a capsule every day. The berries and root (which has a horse like smell), are used to make a supplement which is thought to be similar to ginseng. Inflammation is a marker for disease or discomfort in our bodies. Ashwagandha is reputed to lessen inflammation and pain so has been used for back pain and fibromyalgia.

It is an adaptogen, which means to rebalance and support you in times of stress, stabilising the HORMONE cortisol. Laughter and listening to music you like also lowers cortisol. Ashwagandha works as a general tonic. If you're suffering from "burn out" and adrenal fatigue you could use this supplement to restore you. It is now believed to improve thyroid function in the HORMONAL system. When we are stressed our immune systems can struggle, and this plant supports immune function by increasing white blood cells.

It is thought to enhance BRAIN function by slowing brain cell degeneration, improving memory, focus and reducing anxiety. Could this be worth taking for the early signs of Alzheimer's? Tests on mice at the National Brain Research Centre found that Ashwagandha lowered the amyloid plaques in the BRAIN which are a sign of Alzheimer's.

There have also been promising studies in regard to using this plant to reduce cancer tumours, as it is a powerful ANTI-OXIDANT.

I take it for MENOPAUSE and chronic fatigue syndrome (M.E) to boost my physical and mental state. As it stabilises blood sugar levels it can be helpful to alleviate SUGAR cravings.

Water hyssop (Bacopa monnieri) is an Ayurvedic herb used in Indian medicine and could be useful at the onset of dementia or Alzheimer's as it heightens mental faculties and is said to aid memory and attention.

St John's Wort (Hypericum perforatum) is a herb that is recommended for anxiety and low mood. I have used it alongside herbal remedies mentioned in this chapter for MENOPAUSE instead of HRT. I also take it to alleviate the moodiness I sometimes feel when frustrated by living with M.E (chronic fatigue syndrome). St John's Wort is astringent. It is useful for seasonal affective disorder (SAD) and SLEEP irregularities. The plant chemicals and substances in St John's Wort increase serotonin, the neurotransmitter in the BRAIN linked to contentment. I have known people who have had positive results from using this herb for nerve pain, herpes and headaches. If you are feeling low but are not ready to resort to the antidepressant DRUGS SSRIs, try St John's Wort with a daily walk, a good supplement program and plenty of water. If you start to feel depressed go to your doctor. You may be asked to go to MINDFULNESS sessions or to talk to a psychologist.

Bilberry (Vaccinium myrtillus) contains anthocyanasides which are powerful ANTIOXIDANTS. This herb is excellent at promoting the flow of blood in the body. Along with ESSENTIALS OILS of peppermint and cypress (3 to 5 drops of each in a bath but not taken internally), it will help to alleviate varicose veins.

Feverfew (Chrysanthemum partenium) is a helpful herb if you are suffering with migraines that are related to certain foods and your digestive system. Don't use it if you are pregnant. It's anti-inflammatory so could also be useful for arthritis.

Lesser Periwinkle (vinca minor) has been tested in trials and studies on people with dementia and is given after a stroke to lessen the impact on loss of blood to the brain from a blood clot. Take it as vinpocetine in a supplement.

Vitex (Chaste berry) has an affinity with the pituitary gland in the BRAIN and has a progesteronal action. It is also known as Agnus Castus. It is an excellent herb for a women's HORMONAL and reproductive system and alleviating PMS. Some of the women who suffer with PMS have high levels of the HORMONE prolactin which can lower progesterone levels. Vitex works by inhibiting the release of the follicle stimulating hormone (FSH), and increasing leuteinising hormone. This increases the levels of progesterone so is useful if you are going through the MENOPAUSE without HRT. It's the HORMONE progesterone that drops in the perimenopause. Some companies will combine this herb with others as a menopausal aid. The berries contain essential fatty acids such as linoleic acid. I have taken it alongside Black cohosh and Sage for night sweats and hot flushes during menopause. If you have a history of miscarriage you could take it as preparation for your next pregnancy as it prepares the UTERUS. It is a herb that is also recommended for younger women who suffer with PMS as it helps to rebalance HORMONES. It is useful for mild depression, mood swings, sore, swollen BREASTS, period cramps and bloating.

Black cohosh (Cimicifuga racemosa) is an antispasmodic, mild sedative which can tone the UTERUS. It is helpful when there are low levels of the HORMONE oestrogen. It can be taken for menstrual irregularities, PMS, bloating or for MENOPAUSE. Combined with Vitex (chaste berry), it will alleviate hormonal imbalances which can cause emotional and physical challenges. Avoid it during pregnancy as it is an emmenogogue so it can trigger labour, stimulating contractions in the UTERUS. The Essential oil Clary Sage has this effect too.

False Unicorn Root (Chamaelirium) is also oestrogenic, so can also be used alongside Vitex (Chaste berry) during MENOPAUSE or if you are in the early stages of pregnancy and nauseous. It strengthens and supports the UTERUS. Use a tincture of this herb if you have endometriosis and are concerned about FERTILITY.

Wild Yam (Dioscorea villosa) can be taken as an aid when dealing with infertility, as it increases the flow of reproductive HORMONES and has an affinity with the UTERUS. Along with a drop of ginger ESSENTIAL OIL it can be helpful for nausea during pregnancy.

Squaw Vine (Mitchella repens) is also a tonic for the UTERUS and can be taken in the first three months of pregnancy and after the birth. It is also beneficial for PMT and heavy, painful periods.

Yunnan Bai Yao is a Chinese herb useful if you are suffering with heavy bleeding during the perimenopausal stage. This is a short term temporary treatment. If heavy bleeding continues go to your doctor.

Chai Hu Long Gu Muli Wang benefits the flow of liver energy. In Chinese philosophy and medicine CHI is a fundamental energy present in all living things. The liver is linked to the emotion of anger. Chinese medicine views the MENOPAUSE as a liver and kidney yin deficiency. This herb could be helpful during menopause and for the erratic SLEEP patterns which occur in this stage of life.

Tian Wang Bu Xin Wang is also beneficial if struggling with insomnia and nervous anxiety.

Cramp bark (Viburnum opulus) is helpful to take for dysmenorrhoea or painful periods as it relaxes the smooth muscle in the reproductive area. If you are stressed and your periods have become irregular, this herb can also restabilise.

Scullcap (Scutellaria lateriflora) can be used during pregnancy for restlessness and nerves. It has a calming but fortifying effect on nerves.

Sage (Salvia officinalis) should not be taken during pregnancy as it is an abortifacient. You will also need to avoid it if you have high blood pressure. I have used it for MENOPAUSE, night sweats and hot flushes. Sage is a digestive aid, rebalancing the BOWEL and stimulating hydrochloric acid flow in the stomach. If you have been feeling cold and low after an illness, drink sage tea with a small amount of honey.

Borage (Borago officinalis) is an adrenal tonic so helpful if you feel stressed or run down. It is a galactogogue, so stimulates milk production in the BREASTS in nursing mothers. Take it if you have had a lung infection, bronchitis or pleurisy. It is a diuretic if you suffer with water retention and is anti inflammatory, so could be helpful with other herbs to alleviate rheumatism. You can use it after steroids or cortisone treatment.

Arnica (Arnica Montana) ointment is invaluable if there is bruising and soreness. This is a useful homeopathic treatment for a variety of complaints.

Buchu (Barosma betulina) can be helpful for alleviating infection and inflammation in the URINARY tract and bladder, if you have had cystitis and urethritis.

If you suffer with acne with pustules or scaly, dry skin, **Burdock (Arctium lappa)** could be helpful as it is anti microbial. It has a cleansing, diuretic effect.

Bladder wrack (Fucus vesiculosis) is also diuretic so good for fluid retention before menstruation and lymphatic swelling. It is slightly laxative so along with cascara sagrada can help with constipation. Bladder wrack aids in cleansing the blood and can relieve the SKIN conditions acne, psoriasis and eczema. It contains iodine so rebalances and stabilises under or over activity in the thyroid gland, an important gland in our HORMONAL system. You might see it in products for arthritis and rheumatism.

Comfrey (Symphytum officinale) is also known as knit bone and is helpful when joints, cartilage or tendons have been strained. It is an exceptional healer. I have used it blended with a base oil for muscular back pain and applied it gently to fractures. Internally, it is helpful in healing the gut or BOWEL. It is also an expectorant so may be useful for the lungs and respiratory system. Along with arnica it can reduce bruising. I have also used it with ESSENTIAL OILS on psoriasis and to aid in healing surface skin wounds.

Psyllium husks (Plantago psyllium) turn into a soft bulk to aid in constipation. They improve the peristaltic action of the BOWEL so moving waste and toxins through. You need to drink ample fluid if taking them. You can buy this herb in capsule form.

Yarrow (Achillea millefolium) is an excellent digestive aid relaxing the BOWEL. It could be taken for

IBS along with Slippery Elm, peppermint and elderflower. In combination with the ESSENTIAL OIL cypress, it is helpful for piles and varicose veins.

Dandelion (Taraxacum officinale) can be taken as a tea. It contains VITAMINS A, B and C, Inulin and the MINERAL potassium. It can stimulate kidneys, liver and sluggish digestion, aid in regulating diabetes (supports the pancreas), and is helpful to drink if you have water retention and premenstrual bloating. Effective as a gentle diuretic, I add half a teaspoon of good quality honey to it and buy it in teabags.

Echinacea (Angustifolia or Purpurea) has been in mainstream health news as an aid to preventing and warding off colds, viruses and flu. It is also antifungal, so useful for athletes foot and thrush. You can buy it as a tincture (liquid) or as a product you apply topically to the infected area. I have used it with chamomile and tea tree ESSENTIAL OILS on acne pustules. It works very effectively by boosting T cells in our immune systems. Our skin and tissue naturally contain hyaluronic acid. The bacteria streptococci and staphylococci produce a substance that breaks this natural connection in our tissues. Echinacea works by effectively counteracting this, so that the white blood cells in our immune system fight back.

Golden Rod (Solidago virgaurea) is helpful if you're feeling run down from cystitis and have catarrh and flatulence. I'm currently drinking this as a tea for all three conditions!

Golden seal (Hydratis Canadensis) must not be taken during pregnancy as it stimulates uterine contractions. Avoid it if you have high blood pressure. It brings balance to the digestive system if you're constipated or have diarrhoea. It is a tonic for the UTERUS, improving stimulation there and stabilising heavy periods. Along with Cypress ESSENTIAL OIL it can alleviate haemorrhoids (piles). Like Golden Rod, it can be used for excessive phlegm and sinusitis.

Yellow Dock root (rumex crispus) cleanses the blood and can be used for the SKIN conditions pustular acne, psoriasis and eczema. This herb also gently cleanses the BOWEL when you're constipated, which you want to avoid for optimal health.

Elderflower (sambucus nigra) is another herb used in the battle against colds, coughs and catarrh. It supports elimination of waste and toxins as it makes you sweat. It has an affinity with the kidneys, SKIN and lungs and is a gentle laxative.

Butterbur (Petsites hybridus) was used in the middle ages to treat plague! Today it's an effective remedy for hay fever instead of antihistamines, which can have unpleasant side effects. When this herbal remedy, which contains Zeller's extract, was tested against a range of pharmaceutical hay fever treatments, Butterbur improved symptoms with no serious side effects and worked just as well. You may burp a little if you take it! Avoid it if you're pregnant and don't give it to young children as testing on these groups has not been done. It's not advisable to give it to people with serious liver and kidney diseases.

Liquorice (Glycyrrhiza glabra) is used in Western and Chinese medicine. It is in most oriental herb mixes as it helps to balance SUGAR imbalances. I drink it in herbal teas with other ingredients. It can help heal stomach ulcers and is a mild laxative. If you have cramps from Irritable BOWEL syndrome you could try this herb in a tea with peppermint. It tones the adrenal glands if you're feeling burnt out and exhausted. At times, burn out can also lead to lung infections and this herb is effective as an expectorant for phlegm. Avoid it if you have high blood pressure.

Slippery Elm (Ulmus fulva) soothes the stomach and inflamed BOWELS so could be helpful for hiatus hernia, IBS, colitis (along with Squaw vine) and indigestion. Avoid pharmaceutical anti acid products if possible.

Passiflora (Passiflora incarnata) can be useful for period pains and PMT and is soothing for the BRAIN, mind and neuralgia (pain along a nerve). I take it in teas before bed to help me SLEEP if I'm feeling uptight and tense. If you have relatives with Parkinson's or epilepsy you could recommend this as a tea as it is calming and anti spasmodic.

Valerian (Valerian officinalis) is another calming herb which I take in a capsule before bedtime. Excellent for anxiety and nervousness, I've found it helpful as a SLEEP aid along with herbal teas during MENOPAUSE when sleep can be elusive due to fluctuating HORMONAL levels.

Plantain (Plantago major) has been used for glue ear or infection of the middle ear. It helps to dry up phlegm and catarrhal conditions. It heals the lungs and URINARY tract so helpful for cystitis.

Another herb with an affinity with the URINARY system is **Uva Ursi (Arctostaphylos uva ursi).** It is antiseptic so helpful in healing infections.

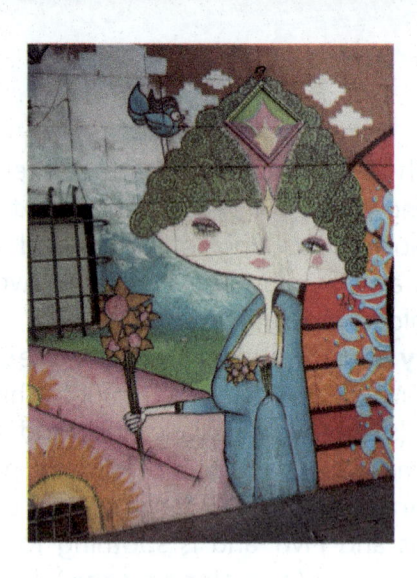

HORMONES

Our endocrine or hormonal system manages over thirty different hormones and regulates metabolism, reproduction and growth development. Hormones are natural messengers that send chemical signals in your body to perform certain jobs efficiently. This is a finely tuned process of signalling. The endocrine glands in the upper body are the pancreas, suprarenal, thyroid, parathyroid and pituitary. They are ductless, which means they secrete directly into the bloodstream or lymphatic system. The endocrine system links into the sympathetic and vagus nerves. Emotional stress can imbalance hormonal signalling.

This next paragraph is for teenagers. Your menstrual cycle runs from the first day of a period or bleed, to the next period. Most women's cycles run for twenty eight days, but this can vary. It is the level of hormones that control the monthly cycle. The main female hormone oestrogen rises at the beginning of the monthly cycle. It

HORMONES

is oestrogen that lines the UTERUS with blood to prepare for a pregnancy. In the middle of the cycle, around day fourteen, ovulation takes place. An egg or ovum is released from an OVARY. The egg will travel down the fallopian tube to the uterus. You're more likely to fall pregnant around three days before, or after, ovulation. If the egg is not fertilised by sperm that has travelled up the VAGINA, you'll have a period. Your periods may stop if you're very anxious or have anorexia nervosa. This is known as amenorrhea. Menorrhagia is the term for very heavy bleeding. Mention this to your doctor if it becomes debilitating. Drink the HERB dandelion in a tea for the IRON and try to avoid becoming anaemic.

You'll either use sanitary pads or tampons which are inserted into the vagina when you menstruate. Choose the lowest absorbency for the flow of blood and change them regularly. Toxic shock syndrome (TSS) is very rare, but can be fatal. TSS occurs when a tampon has been in too long which increases bacteria that produce toxins. If you have any of the following symptoms while using tampons, take it out and tell someone. They include; red eyes, sore throat, feeling dizzy, diarrhoea and vomiting with a high fever.

You can suffer from premenstrual syndrome (PMS), a week or two before your period. You may have difficulty sleeping, so will feel tired and irritable. This could make concentrating challenging. Some women crave SUGAR and carbohydrates before a period so if you're keeping a food DIARY, make a note of it. Your BREASTS might be swollen and sore. You can also have a bloated abdomen or an upset stomach. Cramps can be very painful just before or during your bleed, so take a warm bath and place a hot water bottle on your back or abdomen. They may be linked to an excess of prostaglandins in your system. Read the chapter on HERBS for alternatives to pain killers and to rebalance HORMONES.

If your PMS is severe and affecting your life it is known as Dysphoric Disorder. The 'happy' neurotransmitter serotonin in your BRAIN might be linked to this condition, so you'll feel depressed. You could be advised to go on the birth control contraceptive pill if your PMS is extreme.

Try to EXERCISE during the month, but rest before a period if you need to. Take a high quality multi VITAMIN and MINERAL as most of us are deficient due to poor soil quality and longer storage times for super market foods. The nutrients that may help to lessen PMS are folic acid, calcium, zinc and magnesium, B complex vitamins, vitamin E and D. Eighteen to fifty year olds can take 1,000 milligrams of calcium a day. Avoid too much sugar, salt and ALCOHOL. Read the chapters on HERBS and ESSENTIAL OILS for natural ways to stabilise and fortify your system. In your diary, write down how you're feeling and go to a weekly YOGA, QIGONG or MEDITATION class. Find something to relax you that doesn't involve watching six hours of TV with junk food. Notice when you are stressed.

Oxytocin is a hormone that is released by physical contact, for example, cuddling and orgasm which can initiate a feeling of intimacy. It is also a natural pain and stress reliever. Oxytocin also causes the womb to contract in childbirth and triggers the release of BREAST milk. It also supports the development of neurons in the gut or BOWEL.

The thyroid gland is in the front of your neck, below the larynx. It has two lobes and is connected by a strip called the isthmus. It is involved in many important functions such as nervous system activity, calcium balance, metabolism, energy consumption, temperature and growth and repair. A large percentage of us will have an imbalanced thyroid gland and not realise it. If you are feeling lethargic and have the symptoms listed below, you could ask for a blood test to check your thyroid.

The thyroid produces two important hormones, thyroxin and triiodothyroxine. If you have exophthalmic goitre you will have weight loss, palpitations, anxiety, rapid pulse and digestive upsets and perspire a lot. This is known as Graves' disease or hyperthyroidism. If the thyroid enlarges so that it is visible, it's known as goitre.

The other kind of thyroid imbalance can cause course dry, snake like SKIN. If you are not producing enough of the thyroid hormones and are hypothyroid you might gain weight, feel cold and lethargic, and suffer with constipation. Your pulse rate will be slower. Thyroid issues can also cause depression. These issues may have been triggered by extreme stress, bereavement or an emotional event. Smoking can exacerbate an imbalanced thyroid gland. Hypothyroidism could also be a result of pharmaceutical drugs such as lithium which is prescribed for manic depressive conditions. Cholesterol lowering and heart disease drugs can also adversely affect the thyroid. Countries that add iodised salt inadvertently contribute to hyperthyroidism in the population. Low thyroid function may also be a factor in recurring migraine headaches.

Eat a moderate amount of Brazil NUTS, lentils and legumes once or twice a week (soak them first as they are more easily digested). If you're not vegetarian, include chicken and turkey in your diet, as these all contain the amino acid tyrosine, which, with help from the MINERALS iodine and selenium, will enable you to make thyroxin. ZINC, IRON and magnesium are also important for optimal thyroid function. Use hemp oil as a salad dressing for more of these nutrients. Read the chapter on MINERALS. Include prawns in your diet every month.

However, brassica vegetables (cauliflower, broccoli, sprouts, turnip, suede, kale and cabbage), contain phytates or goitrogens. If you eat them in excess, the phytates in them bind to iodine so that the body cannot use it. Mix up and vary your VEGETABLES. Tea and wheat contain goitrogens which bind to zinc and iron. Include some soaked NUTS in your diet but not in excess, as almonds and walnuts also contain goitrogens. A small handful of nuts a couple of times a week should be sufficient, as they are beneficial for 'healthy fats'.

Cortisol is a hormone that can negatively impact health. Stress and lack of SLEEP can lead to you putting on weight around your waist when the hormone cortisol increases. The adrenalin fuelled flight or fight response links into excess cortisol being released into the blood stream. Cortisol moves glucose into your bloodstream so your muscles can use it, but if your body doesn't use it, fat can then build up around your belly. Your metabolism then slows, and you crave SUGAR. Taking a vitamin C supplement and taking moderate EXERCISE can lower cortisol levels.

Walking briskly for twenty minutes a few times a week is helpful for a myriad of reasons. Plan it into your day and it will become a habit. Try MEDITATION, a YOGA or QIGONG class so that you don't just use a bottle of wine to help you sleep. An oat biscuit or small portion of porridge can help in the evening as carbohydrates can relax you, but eating foods high in protein can be stimulating.

I occasionally use the supplement Melatonin which promotes restful SLEEP and is a hormone that occurs naturally in the body but decreases as you age. Melatonin is produced by the pineal gland. It controls your body clock and works by activating certain types of chemicals in the brain. Try it for twelve weeks, along with a warm, not hot, bath with a few drops of lavender or chamomile dispersed in a teaspoon of milk. If you read a good book before bed that can help, or listen to a guided relaxation meditation from a CD. Don't take Melatonin or use essential oils without advice if pregnant. If you are on HRT it may interact with Melatonin. Some medications can also interact with it so check with your GP or online first. Melatonin is also an effective ANTIOXIDANT and free radical scavenger. Free radicals are rogue atoms that can bounce around your system causing damage to cells. Melatonin has been proven to be twice as efficient as vitamin E in terms of free radical scavenging and helpful as an anti-inflammatory. You can increase your levels of melatonin by eating tomatoes, almonds, cherries and cooking with coriander and cardamom. There are studies indicating that Melatonin assists in anti ageing.

Testosterone is a male hormone but women have it in their system too and it's linked to agility, stamina and muscle mass. Very ambitious, driven, aggressive women tend to have an overload of it. It can cause oily skin.

Gonadotropin-releasing hormone (GnRH) is produced in the hypothalamus in the BRAIN. The hypothalamus is regulated by oestrogen and progesterone and links into our neurotransmitters serotonin and dopamine.

Oestrogen is a female hormone and in excess can slow down the thyroid gland linked to metabolism, can contribute toward water retention and reduce the amount of fat you burn from food. If oestrogen is too low in your system during MENOPAUSE you may have hot flushes, sweats, incontinence, lowered libido and mood swings. If there is an excess of oestrogen you may suffer from premenstrual Tension (PMS), constipation and carry fat around your hips, thighs and buttocks. Excess oestrogen can also cause sore BREASTS, nausea, bloating, VAGINAL bleeding and recurrent vaginal yeast infections.

Oestrogen is lower just before a period and for some women this causes migraine headaches where there is extreme pain, sensitivity to sound and bright light and sometimes, nausea. Women over the age of forty are more prone to migraines.

As women we need both progesterone and oestrogen. If progesterone is low you may suffer with endometriosis, weight gain, hot flushes, heavy periods, post natal depression, infertility or miscarriage - One in four women experience miscarriage. Oestrogen dominance occurs when the levels of the hormone progesterone are lower than oestrogen. The problem is that women are exposed to excess oestrogen from the CONTRACEPTIVE pill and HRT and xenoestrogens in our foods, so the balance is affected. Oestrogen dominance is also linked to an increased risk of stroke and heart disease.

Progesterone helps to maintain bone density, balances blood sugar levels, lifts libido so maintaining desire for SEX, prevents miscarriage, boosts FERTILTY and supports the thyroid gland. If you have an excess of progesterone you may suffer with depression and lethargy.

Fiber binds to Oestrogen and helps remove it from your system. Oestrogen is processed through the liver so reduce alcohol to one unit a day, have a day off from it and take milk thistle as a supplement every few months to support liver function naturally. Take milled flax seed, psyllium husks, konjac fiber and eat plenty of fresh vegetables to increase fiber as well as taking a probiotic such as acidophilus to boost healthy bacteria in your BOWEL, as they metabolise oestrogen too.

Ghrelin is the hormone that lets you know when you're hungry. It will increase when you're stressed, hence the term 'comfort eating'. Very thin people have lots of ghrelin but if you start to gain weight then ghrelin levels drop. Starting a diet will mean that ghrelin levels increase making it challenging to maintain will power when you are tempted by some apple pie. Exercise will keep you preoccupied but research and studies show that swimming in cold water actually increases ghrelin levels. Ghrelin stimulates the release of dopamine, which is a feel good neurotransmitter in the BRAIN by setting off neurons linked to reward and pleasure.

The hormone Leptin is produced in fat cells and its main role is to help in suppressing your appetite. As you put on weight and fat, leptin increases but some people are less receptive to this signalling. If you are obese you may have a lot more leptin in your system and actually feel hungrier when you start eating a meal, then overeat as the fullness messages go unheeded. It's believed that inflammation in the body can disturb leptin levels so make reducing that a priority by increasing OMEGA 3, turmeric and GARLIC supplements, eating a small handful of nuts a few times a week and cooking with chilli, cayenne pepper and herbs. (Avoid too much chilli and coffee if suffering with URINARY tract problems).

    Temperature is now also thought to hinder or help weight loss, so stay slightly cooler to lose weight by turning down the heating and walking in colder weather. Sleep disturbances and sleeping under five hours a night will also affect hormonal balance, so go to bed at 10pm when you can or be in bed at a set time and get up at the same time every day. Oestradiol is our main oestrogen hormone and works in harmony with dopamine to help us sleep and to feel happy and content. Read the chapter on MENOPAUSE for more information about oestrogen.

IRON

Haemoglobin is the protein that transports oxygen from the lungs to the cells. More than half of the body's iron is in its red blood cells as a component of haemoglobin, and low levels lead to less oxygen to the cells. If you have heavy periods and bleeding during MENOPAUSE or menstruation you may become anaemic. This makes you feel lethargic and tired. Haemorrhoids (piles) could also result in blood loss. If you're using an intrauterine device (IUD) as a CONTRACEPTIVE you could become deficient in iron. You need iron levels to be maintained during pregnancy. It can be challenging to consume enough iron daily as 18 mg a day are optimal.

Supplements can cause constipation leading to issues with the BOWELS. There are two kinds of iron. Haeme iron comes from egg yolks, fish and red meat and is easily absorbed. Non haeme iron is from beans, dried fruit and grains. Drink dandelion leaf tea and prune juice if you can, as these are reasonable sources of iron.

Eat poultry (not CAFO, but corn fed and organic if possible). Other sources include; almonds with the skin not blanched, prune juice, spinach and split peas. Take vitamin C as a supplement to aid in iron absorption. Vitamin C is also an ANTIOXIDANT. I use a product called spatone which is a liquid iron supplement containing vitamin C.

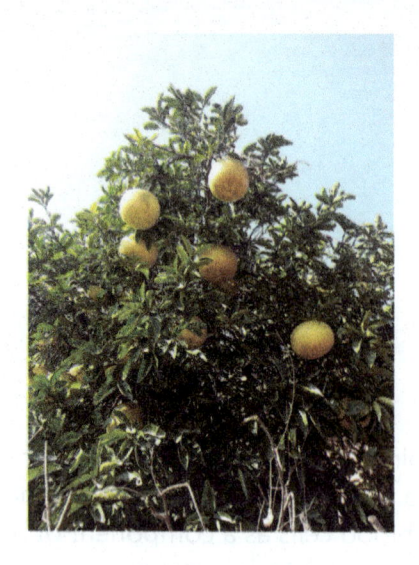

JUICING

Always buy and pick fresh fruit and VEGETABLES for juicing as they'll have higher levels of vitamins, minerals, phyto-nutrients and ANTIOXIDANTS than the pre-packed and processed versions. You'll be able to drink a wider range and greater amount than you would in a single meal so get creative while you increase your body's ability to fight damage from free radicals.

Free radicals are molecules with an unpaired electron which means they are highly reactive. To restabilise themselves they attract electrons from any other molecule, particularly the lipids in our cell membranes, causing damage and creating havoc in our cells, which are the building blocks of good health. ANTIOXIDANTS negate these effects.

Drink mainly raw vegetable juices, due the high content of SUGAR in fruit and add spiralina and wheatgrass to make them even more potent. These two superfoods contain protein and aid the body in eliminating waste. For a zingy taste and an added boost to your digestion add ginger too, and to stabilise blood sugar levels, a sprinkle of cinnamon. You'll feel rehydrated in a matter of minutes. Drink them slowly as soon as you've made them and on an empty stomach, as they contain beneficial digestive enzymes, but will pass fairly quickly through the stomach.

If you're new to juicing you may want to start with carrots, peppers and apples which are full of nutrients and naturally sweet. Add a handful of blueberries as they are now thought to contain a curative substance against malignancy and cancer. Apples lower your chances of dealing with colorectal and liver cancer as they contain pectin which is beneficial for the BOWEL. Eat one when a SUGAR craving starts. Use ripe bananas in your juices occasionally as the brown spots on them contain a substance which combats abnormal cells in the body.

You can then gradually build up the green vegetables and beetroot as you get used to the taste and effect. Drinking raw juice is energising and detoxifying so start with a small amount initially. There are many recipes and combinations to choose from but here are some to get you started. If you are investing in a juicer look at the fusion machines or slow masticating ones and get the best and latest version if you can afford it.

Fruity Ginger

2 whole apples, handful of raspberries, 1 peeled lemon, sliced ginger.

Beety

1 small beetroot, 2 carrots, 1 orange.

Go green

Teaspoon of spirulina, handful of Kale, 1 red pepper, 1 pear.

Red Limey

Half peeled lime, 3 ripe tomatoes, 2 carrots, 1 stick celery.

Capple

2 carrots, 2 apples, half cucumber, 1 teaspoon wheatgrass, 1 teaspoon turmeric.

Melonpower

1 canteloupe melon, 1 banana, grated nutmeg, teaspoon cinnamon.

Leafy

Watercress, parsley, 1 clove garlic, 2 carrots, 1 stick celery.

Pinecabbage

Pineapple chunks, green cabbage, spinach.

JUICING

Grapefright

1 peeled grapefruit, 1 sweet potato, dandelion leaves.

Minty fruit

10 Strawberries, fresh mint leaves, 1 pear, 1 banana.

Cauliapple

Cauliflower florets, 2 apples, 2 carrots, hemp oil.

Sweetie

Mango, blackberries, 1 pear, 1 carrot, cinnamon.

Tomapple

2 ripe tomatoes, 1 apple, red pepper, watercress, broccoli, flax seed oil.

Kaley

Kale, Half peeled lemon, 1 apple, celery, half a cucumber, pinch of turmeric.

Potginger

1 sweet potato, 2 parsnips, ginger, 2 carrots, pinch Cajun spice.

Kiwicabbage

1 kiwi, red cabbage, blueberries, dates, banana.

Asparcumber

1 pear, half a cucumber, 3 asparagus spears, half a stick of celery and squeeze of lemon.

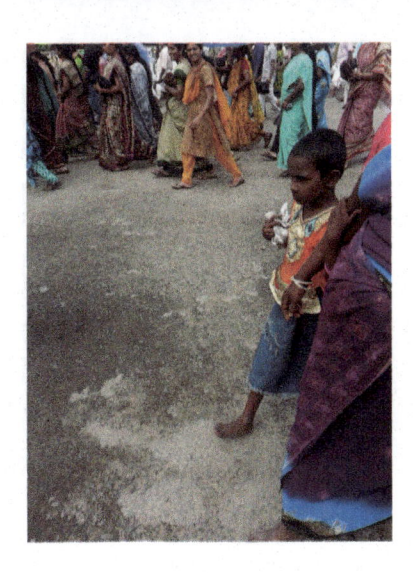

KINDNESS

Kindness, patience and compassion should be an essential part of the syllabus in schools, even if it's just included in a lesson about the religions of the world. Some children are naturally more empathic than others and capable of reading people's facial expressions and body language. They act intuitively and sympathetically. Those children who seem less academic may have other skills and go on to use these in their careers and jobs. Let your child know that they have limitless possibilities if they stay true to themselves, are considerate of others and positive. Encouraging children and teenagers to stop, think and be present, when they're are interacting with others, and to think about how they wish to be treated will help prevent 'one-upmanship' and cruelty. Insist that they ignore and do not become involved with teasing which leads to cyber bullying on social media. Teach your children to abhor and step away from bullying as they develop into kind adults.

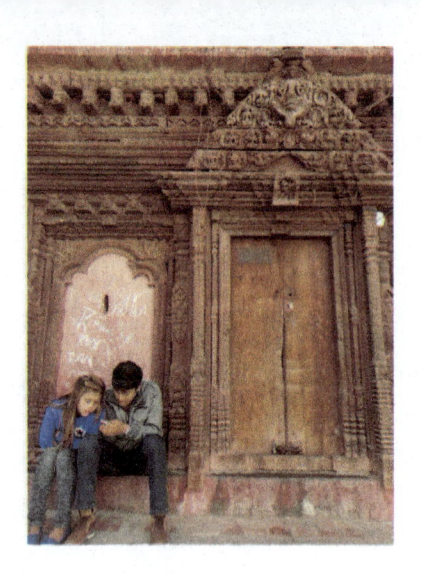

LOVE

Love is patient, love is kind. It does not envy, it does not boast, it is not proud. It does not dishonour others, it is not self seeking, it is not easily angered, it keeps no record of wrongs. Love does not delight in evil but rejoices with the truth. It always protects, always trusts, always hopes, and always perseveres.

Corinthians 13:4

This tiny slice of the bible beautifully sums up love. There are different kinds of love; a mother's unconditional love for a child, the first flush of romantic love and the love we have for our friends

The term Metta comes from the Pali language and translates into "loving kindness". In Buddhism it is a practise where you cultivate this and extend it to everyone. In YOGA the Sanskrit term for this is Maitri.

It can be challenging to love your-self. If we are ill or exhausted, it can feel almost impossible to show kindness to others some days. We have an inner voice

LOVE

that judges and criticises. Be truthful with yourself, caring for your well-being on all levels. Take responsibility for your health and happiness. Only when you accept and truly like yourself (warts and all), just as you are now, will you be able to offer genuine love to other people. Think kindly about yourself. In spite of mistakes and faults, you're essentially a good person. None of us are perfect and needn't pretend we are. Practise being your authentic self whilst attempting to be considerate and kind to others. We all want to be happy and to experience a connection and intimacy with people.

Metta stimulates and plants a seed that grows into wishing everyone good health, freedom from fear and contentment no matter who they are. When I practise Metta, I use the same lines and affirmations. "May I be well, may I be happy, may I be filled with joy and peace". Repeat this in your mind to yourself to begin.

In Metta meditation you then close your eyes and visualise someone you love deeply who has shown you unconditional love. Notice how it feels to focus on imaging this person. You will probably feel GRATITUDE and a deep warmth. The above affirmation now changes to "you".

The next stage of Metta meditation is to visualise a close friend you care about. Observe how that feels to have someone to confide in and laugh with. There is a feeling of connection, sharing, honesty and support with true friends. After this, Metta can seem abstract and difficult but persevere. Next, visualise and imagine someone in your life who is a casual aquaintance. You don't know them well or have strong feelings about them. As you visualise them, send them the same wishes for happiness and health. This can feel strange as you have no personal connection with this person. Metta draws us towards wishing everyone well. The last part of Metta can seem beyond us at times. It involves holding a mental picture of someone we consider an "enemy". They may have deeply hurt or offended us which could still feel like a thorn in your side. When you contemplate them it could bring up physical and uncomfortable sensations. To send this person forgiveness and to wish them well can be extremely challenging, but could ultimately leave you feeling peaceful. Life is short and our egos can take umbrage at perceived offences. Metta does link into the YOGA practise ahimsa or non violence in thought, word or deed. It takes wisdom to know when to discuss an event or situation that upset you. We all want to be treated fairly with consideration.

Get used to the first two stages of Metta meditation initially.

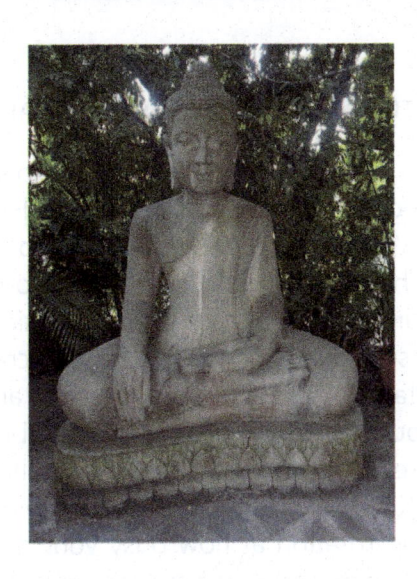

MEDITATION AND MINDFULNESS

Recent studies and research show that in just a short period of time there were profound changes in the structure of the brain's grey matter after thirty minutes a day of meditation or mindfulness practise. The changes, which were highlighted on MRI scans, proved that the hippocampus which is associated with compassion and self awareness had changed and that there was a thickening of the cerebral cortex in areas that link to attention and emotional response.

When we encounter fear or stress it's registered in the thalamus which sends a message to the amygdale, the primitive part of the brain. The amygdale then activates the release of adrenaline. Meditation showed changes in the amygdale indicating that stress and the response would be reduced.

Meditation is a powerful tool in life and should be done most days for optimal effect and benefit, even if it's only for fifteen minutes. There are many different teachers and methods but a simple one is to sit on a chair or crossed legged if you practise Yoga, and lengthen your spine so you're upright. Bring your focus to your nostrils and follow the breath, noticing the sensation of the cool air, or imagine that you're breathing in thick milkshake up straws inserted in your nostrils. Sounds crazy if you've never meditated. Try it. You then just wait and watch to see what your next thought is. It will be about the past or the future and as soon as you notice it you'll 'let it go'. Keep letting go of THOUGHTS and also releasing any frustration or irritation at how busy your mind really is. Notice when there is a gap between your thoughts and your mind stills. As you follow the breath through your nostrils you may find it helpful to repeat in your mind, "I'm breathing in, I'm breathing out", and to say to yourself "I am thinking", when you realise that you're thinking.

Concentration is the first stage of meditation and the results are worthwhile and are now well documented and well known. You'll realise that you're not just your thoughts or emotions and that a 'higher' self can observe them. The more and longer you meditate, the more you become watchful of 'triggers' which are reactions to emotional baggage or old, mental junk you have accumulated. These triggers may bring a negative reaction every time something similar happens in your life, due to pain it caused in your past. Being watchful in your everyday life is the key to a more peaceful life.

Whether you're washing the dishes or on the phone to a difficult relative, stay mindful and aware of reactions. Whenever you can, let go of old hurts and grievances and forgive, because life really is very short. Try to see the other persons' point of view, however impossible it seems at times. Sometimes meditation will entail sitting with

MEDITATION AND MINDFULNESS

yourself on your chair or cushion when you are feeling jaded or disappointed. Accept whatever comes up when you meditate. I have found practising QIQONG very helpful as flowing movements are linked to breath, which is just another way to meditate and move towards a still mind.

Authenticity is important. Being truthful with yourself and acknowledging grief, anger and jealousy will bring what you consider negative, out into the open and the light. Get to the root of those feelings. Sweeping what you consider negative under the carpet and maintaining a fixed smile will ultimately harm you and affect your health. Imagine you are holding your negative emotion in your arms, as if you were cradling a small child and be gentle and compassionate with yourself. Give your full attention to the emotion and notice if you feel it anywhere in your body. The links between what psychologists practise today and mindfulness have become evident. Listen to the inner critic (you), when you meditate and be gentle with yourself. We all make mistakes. As you meditate more and more you'll become aware of when your 'ego' puffs up and becomes indignant. Our ego is not something we need to destroy, as it motivates us in daily life. We just need to keep a watchful eye on reactions and taking things too personally. If you have an insight during a quiet, still moment ask yourself if you need to remove yourself from a situation you cannot change or accept.

We can make plans and goals for the future but it is our presence, our awareness of being the 'witness', to our emotions and being the 'watcher' of our thoughts that bring us moments of joy, contentment and peace. We might then chase down that path, fix our goal as constant, peace and hold spirituality up as our focus and end point. In the end we have to let that go too, and just accept with as much grace as possible the inevitable challenges of life, knowing that whatever is happening is temporary and must be embraced and lived through. Go through your week as if everything that happens has been ordered and arranged by you, for a certain lesson to be learnt.

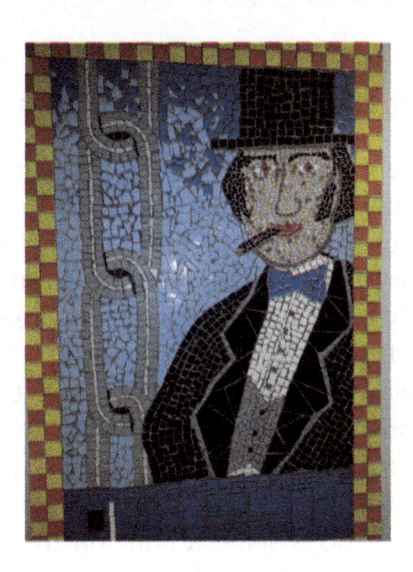

MEN

There is an abundance of decent, funny, caring men in the world. Societal pressures and roles are constantly changing and men have had to adapt to women earning more, being more assertive and expecting men to conform and perform. Clear, honest communication will be helpful in your relationships with men as they're navigating their way through life.

Images, advertising and media bombard us every day and we are all subliminally drawn in and manipulated by this. Look at any magazine, whether it's directed at men or women and you will see women portrayed as scantily dressed, sexual creatures. The TV, social media, YouTube and the internet show clippings and videos of women dancing as if their only goal in life was to be sensual, available and alluring and ready to drop their thongs at the click of a man's fingers.

I recently read an article expressing the attitude that some young men were verbally abusive and disrespectful to the women in their schools, universities and social circles. Is it any wonder when they absorb what is right under their noses in the form of advertising? Pornography may well have its place in today's world but mainstream news recently reported that young girls were struggling to maintain dignity and self esteem due to their teenage boyfriends watching, acting out and expecting sex to be similar to porn they had watched.

Recent cases have come to light regarding abuse decades ago and however disturbing and unsettling this may be, it does shine a light on the way women are perceived and ultimately treated. The bringing to justice of these perpetrators will have led to conflicting opinions.

Educating young boys and bringing them up to see women as equals and people who deserve consideration and KINDNESS will be a start in the process. It will be a battle and an uphill struggle as we all buy into media to some extent. Young girls and women need to be taught self respect and their own value, and to demand this of men who have been brought up to believe that women are inferior. This is not just a cultural problem anymore, it's on our doorstep.

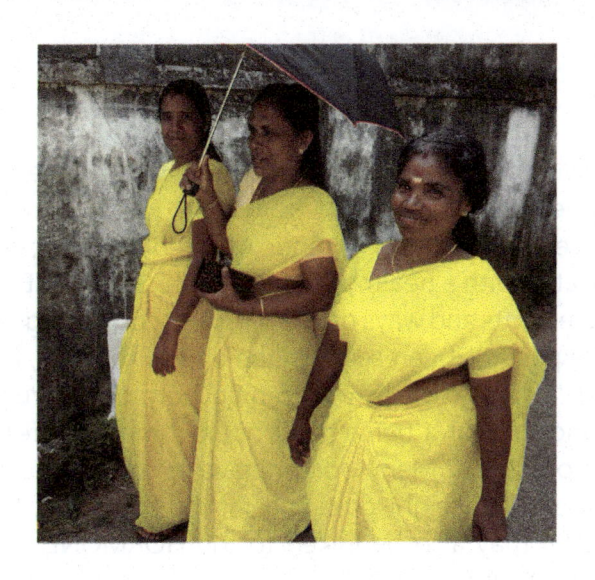

MENOPAUSE

The menopause begins, on average, between the ages of forty eight and fifty two. Levels of oestrogen, the primary female HORMONE may begin to drop around the age of forty five or earlier. The perimenopause is when symptoms may be challenging and your periods start to decrease in frequency. The HORMONE progesterone declines in perimenopause. Once your periods have stopped and you haven't had one for a year, you're considered to be post menopausal. You may need to use CONTRACEPTION for a year after your last period, to avoid pregnancy.

A woman's experience of menopause will vary. If you started in your early or mid forties and suffered with premenstrual tension then you are more likely to struggle. African American may suffer more with menopausal symptoms. Drinking alcohol and smoking will exacerbate symptoms. If you've had your OVARIES removed, patches of HRT, which will be regularly changed, may be prescribed.

Menopause brings a range of symptoms that can be alleviated with a healthy diet, adequate SLEEP, EXERCISE, supplements and ways of lowering and controlling stress. In the past it's been seen as 'the end of the line', a time when 'insane' women with raging hormones struggled to function. For a percentage of us, it may well feel like that some days! Many women have to contend, to some degree, with weight gain and fat redistribution. Excess belly fat may also be linked to the HORMONE cortisol and a lack of SLEEP.

Other problems could include; decreased vaginal mucous secretions and shortening and thinning of the VAGINAL walls, making intercourse painful. Patrick Holford's company Higher Nature, sell an excellent natural lubrication product for this purpose, because if you still have the energy then making love can ensure connection and pleasure for you and your partner, whatever age you are.

Anger, resentment and frustration may come to the surface to be aired if it has been buried. In some Asian and tribal cultures it's seen as a time when a women's workload is lessened and she is regarded as a wise elder. It can be a creative, artistic time when you spend your hours on past times you enjoy. It's a time to nurture, nourish and take care of yourself as you move through another stage of life.

If daily responsibilities start to feel overwhelming, certain situations intolerable and your job and marriage start to suffer, then your doctor may offer you hormone replacement treatment (HRT). A form of HRT contains mare's urine. The process of obtaining this is dubious and to some, unethical, so consider plant options or more ethical forms of HRT, if you become desperate. Some women have experienced HRT as salvation but the risk of BREAST cancer increases once you've been on it awhile. There are three kinds of oestrogen; estradiol, oestrone and estriol. If you decide to take HRT, research your options and start on as low a dose as possible. If you're in your twenties ask for your oestrogen levels now, as they vary in women. You can then attempt to assess how much oestrogen you need at fifty, if you decide on HRT. Some forms of HRT contain oestrogen and meth testosterone. If your ovaries and UTERUS are intact you will probably be offered a combination of estradiol and a progestogen, which is a synthetic form of the natural hormone progesterone. Progestogen has been linked to an increase of fat in the blood and coronary artery spasms.

You may also be offered anti depressants but take these as a last resort. Consider a more natural route and ALTERNATIVES initially, before you make the decision to use HRT, so that you're aware of your choices.

When oestrogen levels drop during menopause, SLEEP can become fragmented which exacerbates your fatigue. Read the section under SLEEP and consider taking melatonin and the herbal remedy Valerian, as you may also be feeling more anxious and emotional. If I feel very anxious and know I'll be in front of a group of people to teach, I'll take a few drops of rescue remedy from the Bach flower essences, which I carry in my handbag.

A lack of internal muscle tone can cause the UTERUS to fall and the URINARY sphincter muscles to lose the ability to contract as well, resulting in leakage of urine (incontinence). Hair may thin and SKIN can lose elasticity and tone. Read the chapter under ESSENTIAL OILS and HERBS for natural remedies. Body hair thins in some women but due to the reversed ratio of oestrogen and androgen (the predominantly male hormone), hair growth on the upper lip and chin may increase.

Another factor of oestrogen levels declining is that bone density is undermined, possibly leading to OSTEOPOROSIS, when bones become 'spongy' and less dense. You may then be at risk from fractures and broken bones. Consider weight training in the gym, as it's never too late to start on a suitable program and it counters OSTEOPOROSIS. You may also have to deal with depression, irritability, impatience, tearfulness, heart palpitations, breathlessness, joint and muscle pain and a slowing down of metabolism.

Lower levels of our HORMONE progesterone initiate perimenopause allowing the hormone oestrogen to become dominant. Natural progesterone is available as a VAGINAL gel. The Chinese nutritional supplement Xiao Yao Wan Plus contains Paeonia which is a female tonic and may help lessen perimenopausal symptoms.

Hot flushes and night sweats are one of the first signs of perimenopause and 80% of women experience them to some degree, for between two and five years. Hot flushes during menopause initiate in the hypothalamus in the BRAIN. When oestrogen levels drop, the follicle stimulating hormone (FSH) and luteinizing hormone (LH) increase. This increase is linked to Gonadotropin-releasing HORMONE (GnRH) surging. Emotions may be erratic and heightened.

The hypothalamus in the BRAIN orchestrates many functions such as body temperature, stress, sleep cycles, metabolism, the menstrual cycle and the autonomic nervous system. The hypothalamus interacts with the neurotransmitters, adrenalin and noradrenalin. Beta endorphins are the BRAIN'S natural mood lifters and regulators. They decrease when oestrogen and progesterone decline. Anger, resentment and frustration may come to the surface to be aired if it has been buried. In some Asian and tribal cultures it's seen as a time when a women's workload is lessened and she is regarded as a wise elder. It can be a creative, artistic time when you spend your hours on past times you enjoy.

After menopause, levels of progesterone decrease dramatically. Try the product Pregnenolone as it is a precursor for progesterone and DHEA (a hormone in our system linked to vitality which declines as we age). Taking Pregnenolone may improve mood and BRAIN function during and after menopause. Joyful Change is another supplement to support changes during this stage of life and is available from Quality Life HERBS.

During menopause the ovaries do not produce so much oestrogen and the adrenal glands take over the production of oestrogen. The adrenals convert androstenadione into oestrone, which is a source of oestrogen after the menopause, as well as producing androgens, which are male hormones linking in to feeling motivated and focused. Body fat also manufactures a small amount of oestrogen and most women put some weight on around this time. EXERCISE will contribute to maintaining healthy adrenal glands.

High SUGAR intake is the bane of our times and as you make your way through your day, eat an apple, pear or small handful of mixed nuts for a snack and avoid the cakes, biscuits and confectionery. I find avoiding junk and sugar difficult in the afternoon, particularly if

I'm filling my car up with petrol as there's an array of sugar as you go to the counter to pay. My solution to this is to keep a small bag of mixed nuts or a banana in the car and a flask of fruit tea with manuka honey in it, to attempt to stave off my cravings. Check the label on some cereal bars as they may be loaded with carbohydrates as puffed white rice and hidden sugar. Sugar will stress the adrenal glands and the pancreas, which produces insulin, resulting in oestrogen not being converted efficiently. The level of adrenal cortical hormone will increase.

Caffeine stimulates the adrenal cortex to produce more adrenalin (which may make you feel more anxious) which leads to the liver breaking down glycogen into glucose. Coffee has its place and it's one of my favourite things in life, but I don't have it after midday and only have a cappuccino once or twice a week, to avoid excessive milk and weight gain. Dairy can also increase mucous. There is research indicating that coffee is helpful for depression, senility and Alzheimer's disease and it does give you a surge if you need to concentrate, but limit it to one or two a morning if you can't give it up.

Phytohormones are substances in plants that encourage the balance of human hormone function in the body. Phytohormones increase 'good' cholesterol, which is the type that removes excessive cholesterol from the blood. Phytohormones keep arteries clear, help prevent cancer and improve blood flow to female organs whilst reducing hot flushes and menstrual problems. These are the foods that contain them so include them in your diet either in soups, stews or teas; sage (reduces hot flushes), liquorice, GARLIC, fennel, green beans, carrots, apples, parsley, rye, oats, red beans, sesame, barley, peas and cherries. Refer to the chapter on RECIPES for ideas on how to include these in your daily diet. Sage and liquorice can be drunk in teas. I particularly like Yogi Tea, who supply a tea called Women's Balance, containing organic HERBS and liquorice. Avoid excessive liquorice if you have very high blood pressure. Pukka teas also have an extensive range which you can substitute for coffee and soda.

The ALTERNATIVES to HRT include; nutritional supplements, HERBS, homeopathy, acupuncture, reflexology and aromatherapy. Read the chapter on ESSENTIAL OILS and blend your own oils to help alleviate symptoms of menopause.

Taking the correct supplements every day will markedly reduce menopausal symptoms. Check the chapters on VITAMINS, MINERALS and VEGETABLES to remind you of the importance and reasons for supplementation as well as a healthy, balanced diet.

The HERBS dong quai, Vitex (agnus castus), black cohosh, false unicorn root, yarrow and motherwort are essential herbs to take during menopause as they can alleviate heavy bleeding, dryness in the VAGINA, restore elasticity and thickness to the vaginal walls, reduce hot flushes and help in normalising HORMONES. Agnus castus supports the pituitary gland in the BRAIN which balances HORMONES. It reduces prolactin levels, so normalising the oestrogen and progesterone ratio and stabilises the happy neurotransmitter dopamine. Agnus castus berries contain health enhancing flavenoids, essential fatty acids such as oleic acid and linoleic acid. These can be taken as supplements in tablet form or tinctures available from a reputable health food shop.

Patrick Holford has a good company called Higher Nature that gives advice and sells high quality supplements.

Ginseng is an adaptogen or normaliser and I take this in a Higher Nature product called Menophase along with other nutrients to alleviate menopausal symptoms. Ginseng is rejuvenating.

Nutrients such as VITAMIN E are hormone normalisers. It has a stabilising effect on oestrogen and reduces hot flushes. When levels of vitamin E are low, the excessive menopausal levels of follicle stimulating hormone and Luteinizing hormone increase exacerbating symptoms. Try starting with 100IU and gradually increasing it to 1000IU. Taking vitamin E can lessen menopausal symptoms such as fatigue, VAGINAL dryness, dizziness, insomnia, heart palpitations and shortness of breath. Take it with selenium as the two nutrients work hand in hand. Along with my multi vitamin and the MINERAL supplement I'm currently taking True food Natural vitamin E from Higher Nature which contains d-alpha tocopherol (a form of vitamin E), and betaglucans.

Vitamin A aids in stabilising blood sugar levels which is essential during menopause. Vitamin A and C can help normalize heavy blood flow during a period. Vitamin C also aids in IRON absorption. The hormone cortisone from the adrenal cortex is sensitive to a vitamin A deficiency.

Heavy bleeding or menorrhagia can occur unexpectedly during menopause. Oestrogen is responsible for lining the uterus with blood and so if an egg is not released that month and progesterone is not produced, the blood flow may be much heavier when you do have a period. If blood flow is constant and excessive, go to your doctor and ask them to check for polyps and fibroids and any signs of UTERINE or cervical cancer. Heavy periods may be linked to your levels of B vitamins being too low, as Oestrogen levels then rise. Too much oestrogen will cause a deficiency in B vitamins. Eat peas, beans and whole grain products for B vitamins along with a B complex supplement. You need at least 50mg of Vitamins B1, B2 and B6 per day. You may be prescribed progestogen the synthetic form of our natural progesterone for heavy bleeds. As an alternative, research wild yam cream instead or vitex or chaste tree in tincture (liquid form). You can help to stabilise hormones to lessen heavy periods.

Wear loose cotton or bamboo clothing, not synthetic fabric, so you stay cool and layer your clothes so that you can shed them in a hot, sweaty moment. Hot flushes can be exacerbated by hot weather, hot drinks, coffee, tea, chocolate and coke. ALCHOHOL and DRUGS and eating large meals too quickly when stressed can also make them worse.

To keep osteoporosis at bay I try to weight train once or twice a week to build bone density. EXERCISE will greatly benefit you, even if it's a walk for half an hour a few times a week. Do more if you can. I currently take a product by Lamberts called Osteoguard for bone health which contains vitamin D, vitamin K, and the MINERALS calcium, magnesium and boron.

If you live in the USA you may be offered the brand name Menest. Premarin is sourced from mare's urine. Premarin is mainly conjugated equine (horse) oestrogen and contains estradiol which is the most potent oestrogen, as well as estriol and oestrone. A dose of only 0.35 a day is linked to good heart health. Much higher doses of HRT may be detrimental to cardiovascular stability as this could increase 'bad' cholesterol. There are many different brands of HRT available. Two of them, Climagest and Clinorette contain Estradiol and progetogen, the synthetic form of the natural hormone progesterone. Ogen, Orthoest and Estrace are from natural sources. Many American women are taking bio identical HRT now.

There's a form of HRT that uses 'bio identical hormones', so similar to our natural body's secretions. These products are sourced from Mexican yam, known as a form of progesterone for many years, and soy. Some women decide to try these alternative creams. Patches and creams that are licensed as bio identical are offered in Britain on the NHS. These contain oestrogen and progesterone not synthetic progestogen. They are applied directly to the SKIN which is thought to be more effective as they are not processed through the liver. The brands are Hormonin, Estrogel and Estraderm. Recent research in France points to evidence that these bio identical products that contain oestrogen and progesterone could protect women from cancer, heart attacks and dementia. Britain now has access to a progesterone pill branded as Uterogestan. The long term effects of these bio identical products are not yet known.

MINERALS

Many of us are deficient in essential minerals due to the depletion of farmers' soil and eating too much processed and packaged food. Nutrients enhance and assist each other, so eat a varied diet and take a well rounded and formulated multi vitamin and mineral supplement. You can be tested to find out which nutrients you are deficient in.

We need the macro minerals calcium, potassium, phosphorus, magnesium and chloride for optimal health. Iron, zinc, sodium, manganese and chromium are also important in the correct amounts for the body to assimilate and utilise them.

Selenium is a vital, non metallic element needed in trace amounts and is a powerful ANTIOXIDANT. It protects you from heavy metals such as mercury, lead, cadmium and arsenic. It is in the enzyme glutathione peroxidise which reduces damage in cells and in the enzyme deiodinase, which is required for the production of hormones in the thyroid gland which regulates metabolism. It must be taken with vitamin E. The best food source is Brazil NUTS but eat cashews, tuna, salmon and white fish to get your selenium. Wild Alaskan salmon is lowest in heavy metals. Wheat germ, wholemeal bread and bran also contain selenium but can cause dietary intolerance or sensitivity in some people.

If you lack vitamin D because you never expose your skin to sunlight, you may have a calcium deficiency. If you take corticosteroid drugs, the contraceptive pill or diuretics to flush out fluids, you may also be lacking in this vital VITAMIN.

Coeliac disease, lactose intolerance and low stomach acid may impair calcium uptake. If you're taking a calcium supplement for bone density, ensure it contains Boron too, which you can absorb naturally from prunes, almonds and dates. Cheddar, Edam cheese and sardines are good sources of calcium. The ratio of calcium to Phosphate should be 1:1. Your DNA contains Phosphate and as ATP adenosine triphosphate, it is needed as the energy molecule metabolically.

If you're vegan you may have low levels of calcium, as it's found in dairy produce, so may need to supplement it along with vitamin B12. Potassium is important for the functioning of muscles and nerves, helps control blood pressure, takes oxygen to the brain, helps eliminate body waste and is needed for the secretion of Insulin by the pancreas. Potassium and sodium as a team maintain the acid base balance of the blood.

The metabolism of carbohydrates is partly dependant on the minerals chromium, magnesium and potassium so a lack of them may contribute to fatigue which is a factor in MENOPAUSE and M.E.

Magnesium is needed for many different processes in the body. Read the chapter on OSTEOPOROSIS. Include lentils, a small amount of wild rice, almonds, split peas, bean sprouts and spinach in your diet every week to ensure you get enough. If you're not vegetarian, chicken and beef are options to increase magnesium but buy organically reared or corn fed and free range to

MINERALS

avoid the alarming and detrimental effects of ingesting growth hormones and antibiotics that are fed to animals. Consider where they came from and exactly what you're putting into your system before you serve them up. Ensure you drink enough water and herbal teas before meals, not straight after, to avoid dehydration.

Potassium is also linked to energy so take levels of between 2,000mg to 3,000mg a day. Buy fish (wild and fresh if you can) two to three times a week and eat bananas, avocados, oranges and peas for potassium.

Chromium helps to stabilise blood sugar levels by working with insulin secreted from the pancreas. You can take up to 200mcg if you are obese or have blood sugar problems. Alongside a reduction in junk food and with EXERCISE it will help to build muscle and burn fat. Chromium is essential for glucose, insulin and fatty acid metabolism. It declines as you age and can be helpful on a weight loss program. Check your multi supplement to see if chromium picolinate is used, as this is the best form to take. You can take up to 200 mcg a day of chromium picolinate or polynicolinate, but not chromate.

NUTS

Eating a small amount of nuts a few times a week will improve your health and assist you if you're on a weight loss program. Nuts are fairly high in calories, so it's best not to eat too many. They contain VITAMINS and MINERALS, 'healthy fat' and an amino acid called l-arginine. Amino acids are the building blocks of protein. Nuts are nutritious powerhouses and are filling and satisfying, as well as protecting you from degenerative diseases such as cancer and heart complaints. Include Brazil nuts, walnuts, hazelnuts, macadamias, cashews and pecans in your weekly food shop instead of packaged processed food. Macadamia nuts contain decent amounts of monounsaturated oleic acid, vitamin B1, magnesium and manganese. Almonds are actually the seed of the fruit of the almond tree. They contain the MINERALS calcium, IRON, ZINC, magnesium, manganese, potassium and VITAMIN E. Include a few almonds in your daily diet with berries and plain, natural yogurt or sprinkled on top of a salad. They are alkaline forming like vegetables, which is beneficial for health. You can soak them overnight so that they are a little easier to digest.

They're ideal for everyone to snack on, but check for nut allergies if offering them to children you don't know. Nuts are particularly beneficial if you're struggling with MENOPAUSE and craving sugar.

OMEGAS

The two essential fats are linoleic acid and alpha-linolenic acid. The two essential fish oils are EPA and DHA. They are in what is known as 'cis' form, a chemical configuration which means they slot into our bodies and cells to prevent inflammation and disease. If vegetable oils are fried this perfect 'cis' chain is distorted and not only becomes unusable, but is actually toxic to our systems.

Most of us have enough Omega 6 in our diets but many of us are deficient in the essential fatty acid Omega 3. Our bodies don't produce OMEGAS so to get them, it's important to take these as a supplement and to eat oily FISH a few times a week. They are very important for cell membranes, our BRAIN and our mental health, as well as our cardiovascular systems and hearts. Heart attacks can kill women too but the symptoms may be different. The beginning of one can feel like indigestion and like a large ball going slowly down the oesophagus. Other signs are squeezing motions racing up the spine and under the sternum, branching into both jaws. If you think you're experiencing a heart attack, call 999 emergency then lie down after taking an aspirin.

Omegas also ensure the smooth running of our nervous systems, assist in joint mobility and aid in weight loss. We obtain EPA and DHA from oily fish such as sardines, mackerel and salmon. Tinned tuna doesn't have much Omega 3 in it. Have fish two or three times a week, not every night, as there are issues with what farmed fish are fed and the accumulation of heavy metals and pollutants in sea fish end up in our tissues. Buy fresh wild Alaskan salmon when you can.

Omega 3's act in the body to produce vital messengers called prostaglandins which contribute to destroying cancerous cells. Alpha-linolenic acid is found in hemp, flax and chia seeds. Flax oil is the most balanced of these in terms of omegas so add it to salads or put a teaspoonful in smoothies. I put a small amount in my soup and natural yogurt just before I eat it. If you eat flax seed or chia the ALA in it needs to be converted to the beneficial EPA and DHA. Milled flax seeds are a tasty topping on porridge with a sprinkling of cinnamon.

The protein profile of Hemp is similar to human blood. This can also be taken in oil form and I use it to make salad dressings with garlic, lemon juice and balsamic vinegar and parsley. Hemp is incredible and worth adding to your diet as it contains all essential amino acids, two key globulins, albumin and edestin, which is similar to protein in the human body so can repair DNA. It contains Omega 3 and 6 in the ideal ratio for optimal health. Hemp seeds contain IRON, magnesium and ZINC helping to reduce cravings and improve memory function. If you dislike fish, or you're vegetarian, start taking algae as a supplement as it is a viable alternative.

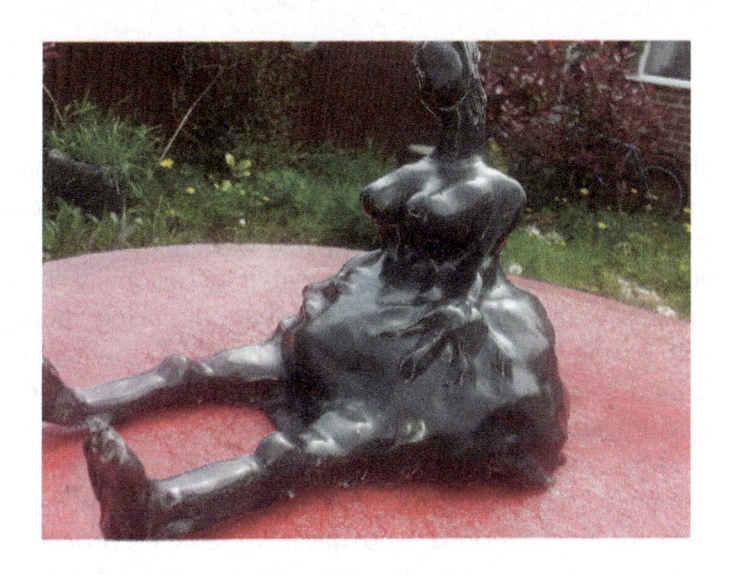

OSTEOPOROSIS

Our bones are constantly dissolving and regenerating throughout our lives. The cells osteoclasts dissolve bone and osteoblasts replace it with new bone. When we develop osteoporosis the internal part of the bone becomes spongy and we're more likely to experience a fracture or break. Bone mass starts to decline before the menopause in our mid thirties but is accelerated around the time of menopause. Weight bearing exercise from a young age will offset and prevent osteoporosis from developing in later life

A diet excessively high in salt, fibre and protein will draw calcium from your body. Fibre from fruit, vegetables and milled flax seed is beneficial for a healthy bowel and very helpful if you're trying to lose excess weight, but if you overdo it, it will prevent your intestines from absorbing calcium.

Too much protein in your diet will result in ketosis and an acidic body. Meat, excessive coffee consumption and alcohol are acidic and fruit and vegetables are alkaline. An acidic system can eventually lead to disease. Spinach contains high levels of oxalates that bind calcium so your body can't absorb it, so eat it occasionally. I've been experimenting with my blender and making soups with spring greens, cabbage, bok choi (high in vitamin C) and kale. Add kidney beans to soups and stews for calcium and colour.

Milk and cheese are not the only options when it comes to absorbing the MINERAL calcium. Include sardines, figs, almonds, kelp, green vegetables, broccoli, carrots and sesame seeds to increase your intake of calcium to keep bones healthy and strong. High quality plain, natural yogurt with no added fruit or sugar is beneficial in small amounts but commercial dairy may contain xenoestrogens, bovine growth hormones which can disrupt hormonal balance. Avoid fruit yogurts daily and have them as a dessert once a week.

Drinking excess milk will lead to weight gain due to the high fat content and may increase mucous. If you are lactose intolerant this could be problematic. The enzyme lactase digests lactose in milk and as we age this decreases, making lactose intolerance very common. If you happen to be one of those women and you drink milk, studies show that you are at risk of developing ovarian cancer. Galactose is a sugar in lactose which can adversely affect fertility and in predisposed women is toxic to ovaries. Try almond milk as an alternative and avoid drinking soya milk every day, as it's the main genetically engineered crop, along with corn.

High levels of adrenaline in our systems from constant, prolonged stress will reduce and undermine bone efficiency. If you smoke, it can reduce your bone mass by around 20% as smoking affects the balance of female hormones, lowering oestrogen. Smoking and alcohol also affect blood sugar levels which you need to maintain at a constant level.

If I have porridge oats a few times a week I make it with cinnamon, for its' blood sugar stabilising effects, with half a teaspoon of manuka honey and almond or coconut milk with a small handful of blueberries and a few walnuts and almonds. The effect of genetically modified food on our systems is unknown, but massive levels of toxic pesticides are used in the growing and proliferation of soya and corn. Some advocate taking soya supplements during menopause as it's a phytoeostrogen. I have decided to try other herbal alternatives. I have stopped eating tofu and drinking soya milk as research is pointing towards the heightened benefits of fermented soya in the form of tempeh, and miso soup. Include natto and kimchi in your diet. They can be found in Asian stores and are beneficial. Oriental women don't seem to suffer as much in the menopause because they include them in their diet. The company Clearspring make a miso soup with sea vegetables and it is quick, convenient to make, and tasty.

A woman over fifty requires 1200 mg of calcium every day. Adequate levels of stomach acid are required along with vitamin D to absorb the calcium. We need twice the amount of magnesium to calcium for healthy bone formation. Magnesium is essential for burning glycogen for fuel and for muscle contraction. Take it in the aspirate form.

If you eat too much meat and protein, which creates acid in your body, you will be losing your calcium stores. If you eat an extra 10 grams of protein you will lose

100mg of calcium. Eat more vegetable soups, stews and salads and reduce red meat and dairy.

Don't buy commercial fruit yogurts as they're loaded with sugar. Buy a good quality natural, plain yogurt and have a few tablespoons a day with linseeds and sunflower seeds.

If you can't give up coffee or wine, ensure that you only have one or two cups of coffee before midday and two days a week alcohol free. For optimal health, drink red wine and only have one small glass a few nights a week, so that your liver can remove toxins from your system.

The best way to take a supplement is to invest in a good multi vitamin and mineral as the correct levels of nutrients need to work synergistically, so the science has already been done for you. I buy Solgar and Higher Nature as I greatly respect Patrick Holford, a renowned nutritionist. If you are diagnosed with brittle bones you will be advised to take an additional supplement and to be effective this should include calcium citrate in conjunction with Vitamin C, D, magnesium, copper, manganese, silicon and boron.

Magnesium increases calcium and vitamin C absorption so enhances your body's ability to retain it to form bone. Sixty percent of our body's magnesium stores are contained in the bones of the vertebrae, thighs and wrists. Magnesium also helps to convert vitamin D to an active form, enabling calcium to be absorbed effectively. Avoid calcium carbonate in supplements as this is basically chalk and not absorbed well. Calcium citrate is the better option so check the labels on your supplements.

If you eat instant, processed food and consume fizzy drinks you will be taking in far too much phosphorus.

OSTEOPOROSIS

The balance of phosphorus to calcium should be equal for bone health so limit packaged, processed puddings and meat and avoid large quantities of cottage cheese. Taking 3mg a day of the trace element boron will increase the amount of oestradiol, an oestrogen hormone in the blood and will greatly reduce the amount of calcium excreted in your urine. HERBS such as horsetail and alfalfa are often used to treat osteoporosis.

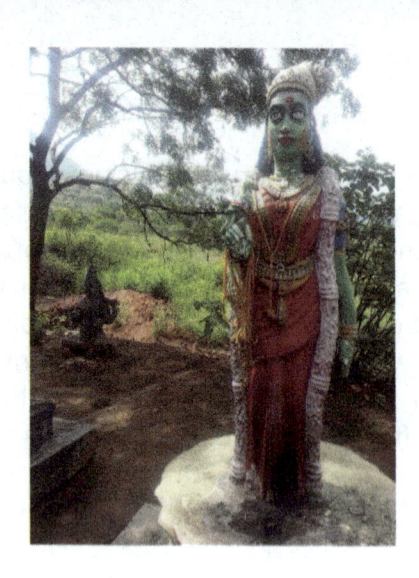

OVARIES

The two ovaries are situated on either side of the UTERUS in the lower abdomen. Every month they release an egg or ova and the HORMONES oestrogen and progesterone. As part of a women's menstrual cycle, the egg grows in a small sac inside the ovary. This is called a follicle and most of the time it splits open to release the egg. This generally occurs once a month. If the follicle doesn't open, a cyst can form from the fluid inside. These are harmless.

There are a few different kinds of cysts and they are nothing to worry about and fairly common. If a large cyst moves and twists and blocks blood flow to an ovary, it can damage it. This is known as ovarian torsion and is fairly rare.

If a cyst ruptures you will experience pain and bleeding and will need medical aid immediately. This rarely happens. If you have the symptoms listed below you can be referred to a specialist for an ultrasound. This uses high frequency sound waves so that an image of the internal pelvis can be examined. CT scans and MRIs are other technological tests to see internal images. If you're diagnosed with desmoids or cyst adenomas and are hoping to conceive, your FERTILTY won't be affected. Cysts tend to occur more in postmenopausal women.

Polycystic ovarian syndrome (PCOS) is a debilitating condition which may be hereditary and genetic. The ovaries will contain a large number of small cysts. There is an imbalance in the female sex HORMONES with PCOS, which can cause problems with weight gain, menstruation, infertility, miscarriages in the first trimester (12 weeks), acne and excessive facial hair. Depression may also become a factor and the symptoms will continue to exacerbate it. Miscarriages are more common in obese women and are caused by a variety of reasons. Seventy five percent of miscarriages occur in the first trimester.

Insulin, the hormone secreted by the pancreas gland, moves SUGAR from the blood stream to the liver to be converted to fat. If you have PCOS and you're insulin resistant you'll store fat too efficiently. Glucagon is the HORMONE which converts stored sugar in the liver (glycogen) and stored fat into sugar that the body uses for energy. Insulin resistance can lead to type 2 Diabetes and cardiovascular disease.

About ninety percent of ovarian cancer cases are made up of epitheal tumours. Cancer can be hereditary or genetic and you can ask to be tested if it is in your family. The chances of being diagnosed for ovarian cancer increase after MENOPAUSE, the age of sixty and if you are overweight. White women seem to have higher incidences of it as opposed to Hispanic and black women. You may have a higher risk if you have not given birth, had a later MENOPAUSE, taken HRT, started your periods before the age of twelve and gave birth to your first baby after the age of thirty.

The main symptoms of ovarian cancer are: needing to urinate more often and urgently, constant bloated belly and abdominal discomfort and pain, feeling full quickly when you eat and finding it difficult to eat, losing weight rapidly and feeling exhausted. You might also suffer with indigestion, flatulence and nausea or have alternating constipation and diarrhoea. Other symptoms are back pain and discomfort. It is the fifth most common type of cancer. There may be blood spots after intercourse or an unpleasant smelling discharge. An ovarian tumour will rest on the abdomen or in the fold connecting the stomach to other internal cavities. The blood test CA-125 screens for ovarian cancer but is not 100% effective. You may be offered a hysterectomy or removal of the ovary if it is tested and not benign. I have a client who used frankincense and cypress ESSENTIAL OILS in a daily bath to relax her during her treatment. We used breathing and relaxation techniques every day.

Regular EXERCISE, a varied diet with VEGETABLES and ANTIOXIDANTS and ways of keeping stress at bay, will offset your chances of ill health.

PRODUCTS

Buying and using products is a form of reward and pleasure for women, leading to heightened self esteem and relaxation. For centuries we have bathed and luxuriated and slathered ourselves with all manner of lotions and liquids. It's the feel good factor linked to the belief that we look more attractive. Beauty is more than SKIN deep and comes from an inner radiance, when a woman is content and confident. Balanced self esteem is a part of our mental and emotional health, just guard against vanity and constantly comparing yourself to other women. You'll have your own style and kind of beauty, so embrace that.

We use make up to enhance our looks and although it is a kind of mask, it can give us confidence and is part of our creativity. For some women, putting on their face is a comforting ritual. Begin to think about exactly what you are using in the form of products. Studies have shown that lipsticks can contain extremely high amounts of heavy metals like lead and cadmium. You swallow a certain amount of lipstick when you eat and drink. Heavy metals are toxic and are stored in BREAST tissue and the organs through your body. Invest in organic, natural products when you can. Check the labels on exfoliates or scrubs for micro beads as these do not break down when washed down your sink. Plastics such as these will take hundreds of years to disintegrate. They adversely affect the Environment. Micro beads will soon be phased out.

Avoid using talcum powder. This can cause ovarian cancer if used over a long period. If you know someone who puts talc on their tampons or underwear or in the genital area, share this with them and inform them of research.

Nature provides a huge and varied amount of substances that we can use ourselves. I regularly make skincare products with jojoba oil and ESSENTIAL OILS. You may be surprised as to how many wonders of nature are being used in products. Cochineal bugs are pulverised into a red powder to make some lipsticks deep red. Ambergris is a waxy substance that whales excrete in bowel movements and vomit. Amazingly, it's mixed into perfumes to enable the aroma to linger for longer. Perfumers and 'noses' (people who sniff and blend fragrances as a job), are experimenting with more and more unusual ingredients. The boundaries are now blurred as to what is a feminine or masculine scent, as gender sensibility becomes more fluid and open.

Fish scales contain a substance called guanine which is included in some cosmetics to make them sparkly. Snails excrete glycolic acid and elastin, substances that have been inadvertently used through the ages and are now part of skin care products which enhance cell turnover for smooth skin. Lanolin also moisturises the skin effectively and comes from sheep's wool.

There aren't many products out there that are 100% organic but more and more companies are attempting to source and use organic ingredients and include them in their ranges. Check the chapter on CHEMICALS and

PRODUCTS

as much as you can, avoid using them on your skin and hair. Companies to try are Origins, Aveda, Green people, Neal's Yard and the Organic Pharmacy. Go to uk.100percentpure.com. Research new ethical, organic brands to try as entrepreneurial women are designing exciting, effective products.

One way to peel a group of teenage girls off their phones and social media is to arrange a natural product party. Go online for some of the ingredients and to get recipes. Go to SharAmbrosia.com, Kalyx.com and Homemade-beauty.com. Gather your group with towels, tissues, flannels and bowls of boiled water and a bin. Whisk, create and blend cleansers, toners, exfoliates, moisturisers and masks using plain yogurt, honey, oat flakes, lemon, witchhazel, egg whites and Kelp (fucus vesiculosis). Include ESSENTIAL OILS but only use a drop or two as they are powerful and concentrated, so always dilute them.

The following face and body products are beneficial, ethical, nurturing and effective.

Green people sunscreens.
Green tea Oil Free Hydration SPF 30.
Neal's Yard Wild Rose Moisturising SPF 30 facial cream.
Avalon Organics Vitamin C Renewal Moisture Plus Lotion SPF 15.
Neom Luxury unwind skin treatment organic bath and body oil with Bergamot and Lavender
DHC Deep Cleansing Oil with olive oil and vitamin C
Huni Manuka Honey every day soap in Kowhai with Propolis and Royal Jelly
Elemental Herbology Biodynamic facial soufflé
Dr. Alkaitis organic nourishing treatment oil.

A TO Z MINI-GUIDE TO WOMEN'S HEALTH

TSI-LA natural eau de parfum with natural extracts
Saaf organic ultimate moisture face serum
Inika mineral blush in kiss kiss, playful and vavavoom
Saaf organic eraser body oil for scar tissue
Jo Wood organics everyday cleansing mousse
Origins organics body pampering massage oil
Green people triple action cellulite lotion
Joshi's Holistic skincare body treatment
Ila cleansing bath salts
Bamford organic bath oil with geranium
Neals yard remedies Grapefruit and Juniper gel
The Organic Pharmacy self tan
Liz Earle superskin moisturiser
The Organic Pharmacy sheer tint in bronze glow
Athena seven minute liftwith avocado, orange and sweet almond
Nuxe serum merveillancewith mimosa seed oil, oak extract and calendula
Non tox-PP3 ultra potency lip plump with plant extracts and menthol
Face Boutique Peachy clean foaming face wash
Chantecaille Rose eye makeup remover

QIGONG

An ancient practise from China, which utilises breath and movement with MEDITATION, is as applicable now as it was centuries ago. Women endure through hectic timetables, responsibilities and efforts to nurture and maintain relationships. We run homes, nourish and love families and hold down demanding jobs. It's no wonder exhaustion sets in at times and we struggle to pull everything together.

There will come a time when you have spare time just for you. If you decide to start this profound practise now, ten minutes a day will be beneficial if that's all you have. I started qigong at forty nine because I felt it would be a way of moving mindfully towards my seventies. I have found it invaluable in staying calm and relaxed during MENOPAUSE.

It's satisfying, grounding and centring and as I have had to tune in to my energy levels from living with chronic fatigue syndrome for thirty years, it has proved to be a helpful tool. Through simple movements and concentration, it encourages tension to leave your body and anxieties to dissipate gently from your psyche. It subtly clears negativities and allows you to let go of unhelpful patterns in your body and outdated, unhelpful thoughts and traits.

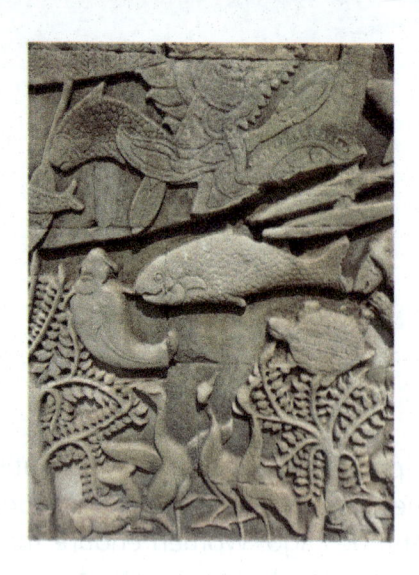

RECIPES

Sicilian Caponata

2 tbsp cold pressed Olive oil
1 large aubergine cut into large cubes
1 red pepper, seeded, cut into large cubes
2 tsp dried oregano
Half tsp dried chilli flakes
2 sliced garlic cloves
1 small finely chopped onion
Finely chopped parsley
Handful of mint leaves
4 ripe tomatoes cut into large cubes
250g pitted green olives
4 tbsp drained pickled capers
2 tbsp apple cider vinegar

Heat the oil in a large pan. Add the aubergine, pepper, oregano and chilli and cook over medium heat for 5 minutes, stirring occasionally. When browned, add the garlic, onion, most of the parsley and mint and cook for another 3 minutes. Add the remaining ingredients and cook for 20 minutes. Serves 2.

Taken from *Green Kitchen travels* by David Frenkiel and Luise Vindahl.*

Broad bean and pea puree

200g of frozen or fresh broad beans
200g of frozen pea
6 tbsp extra virgin olive oil
2 shallots, sliced
3 gloves garlic, sliced
Juice of 1 lemon
Mint leaves
Salt and pepper
300g natural or Greek yogurt

Steam the beans and peas until cooked
Heat 2 tbsp of olive oil and fry the shallots and garlic
Blend them in a blender with peas and broad beans and remaining ingredients apart from yogurt
Add yogurt and blend again briefly.
Drizzle with olive oil.

Taken from *House and Garden* May 2013*

Warm Salad of Roast Butternut Squash with Pine nuts and Feta

450g Butternut squash peeled and chopped

2 red onions peeled and chopped
100g feta cheese crumbled
50g Pinenuts toasted 5 minutes
2 Tbsp Olive oil
2 tsp Balsamic vinegar
2 Tbsp chopped
Salt and black pepper
150g baby spinach

Oven 180C/250F/Gas 4
Place the squash and red onion on a baking tray and coat with olive oil and salt and pepper.
Cook in hot oven for 40 minutes adding the sage and for the last five minutes. Remove from the oven sprinkle balsamic vinegar. Serve on pile of spinach topped with feta and pine nuts.

Taken from *Om magazine* www.ommagazine.com*

Roasted Tomato and Chickpea Curry

1 kg ripe tomatoes
80ml olive oil. Tin chickpeas
6 cardamom pods, crushed
Half tsp fennel seeds
Half tsp black mustard seeds
6 cloves and 2 star anise
1 small dried chilli
1 tsp ground cumin and black pepper
1 tsp ground coriander and fresh leaves
Half tsp turmeric
250 ml coconut milk
1 medium onion

RECIPES

3 cloves grated garlic
1 tbsp fresh grated ginger

Preheat oven to 180C/350F, gas mark 4.
Place tomatoes in roasting tin. Drizzle half oil, sprinkle salt. Roast for 10 minutes. Take half tomatoes to chop and peel. Heat frying pan and add spices and chilli. Heat oil in saucepan add onion, garlic and ginger for 10 minutes.
Add spices and fry for 2 minutes.
Add some tomatoes and coconut milk and simmer for 15 minutes.
Add the chickpeas and 12 reserved tomatoes and simmer gently for 10 minutes
Serve with naan bread and yogurt.

Taken from *New Feast by Greg and Lucy Malouf.**

Broccoli, celery and dill soup

2 tbsp coconut oil
1 clove garlic, crushed
1 spring onion, chopped
Quarter tsp caraway seeds
Half tsp ground coriander
700ml boiling water
3 sticks celery, chopped
Finely grated zest and juice half lime
100g broccoli and 100g spinach
Quarter of an avocado
6g dill
Quarter of tsp pink Himalayan salt

Heat 1 tbsp of coconut oil in pan. Sauté the garlic and spring onion with the caraway seeds and ground coriander for 2 minutes, then add 100 ml of boiling water. Add the celery and lime zest, juice.
Leave to simmer for 7 minutes. Add 400 ml of water and return to boil. Add broccoli, remaining water and spinach leaves. Transfer contents to a blender. Add the avocado, dill, salt and 1 tbsp coconut oil and blend until smooth. Serve hot.

Taken from *Marie Claire* magazine. February 2015.*

Harissa with Roast Vegetables and Quinoa

2 peeled plum tomatoes for Harissa
Quarter tsp cayenne pepper
1 tsp cumin powder
1 tsp coriander powder
1 clove garlic
Dash of vinegar
Roast vegetables
225g quinoa and 860ml water
10 cherry tomatoes
1 medium carrot and onion, sliced
1 courgette, cubed, 2 tsp of olive oil
1 red pepper, sliced

Place these ingredients in a blender to make the Harissa.

Place all the vegetables on a baking tray. Lightly drizzle with olive oil. Bake in a preheated oven 180C/350F/gas 4for 50 minutes. Shake tray twice to turn vegetables Rinse quinoa. Place in saucepan with water. Bring to boil

RECIPES

cover and simmer for 13 minutes. Serve with vegetables and Harrisa.

Taken from Patrick Holford. Fatburner Diet.*

Crunchy Thai salad

Small white cabbage, shredded
8 runner beans, sliced
1 chopped tomato
1 chilli, finely chopped
Juice of 2 limes
1 tsp fish sauce
1 tsp apple juice
Handful of peanuts, crushed

Combine all the ingredients in a large bowl and toss well. Omit the chilli if you dislike spicy food.

Cheesy Leek and cauliflower mash

2 large leeks washed and sliced
1 cauliflower, chopped
Half a white onion
2 cloves garlic
Sea salt and pepper to taste
Sour cream and knob of butter
Chunk of cheddar cheese
Tsp Turmeric

Steam the vegetables for 5 minutes. Lightly fry the garlic in butter until soft. Put into a food processor or blender and add seasoning and sour cream.
Grate cheddar cheese and sprinkle on top
Put dish in.preheated oven to melt cheese 180C/350F/gas4
Not vegetarian? Try it with fried bacon or monkfish.
Omit the cheese for vegans and add shitake mushrooms.

Beany salad

Plateful of Rocket
Swiss chard, shredded
White turnip, 1 carrot
Butterbean
Aduki or black beans
Kidney beans
Green beans.
Goats cheese

Arrange the rocket on a plate and add dressing of choice. Grate the turnip and carrot. Steam for 2 minutes with the chopped green beans, chard. Leave to cool then add to salad. Add a cupful of mixed, canned or soaked and precooked beans Toss the veggies and add small chunks of goat's cheese. If you are vegan top with peanuts or macadamia nuts.

Courgette and pumpkin chips

Splash of olive oil

RECIPES

Chilli powder, quarter tsp
2 large courgettes,
Pumpkin or swede chipped
1 egg

Whisk the egg and olive oil with splash of water and chilli powder (or black pepper). Coat the courgette and swede chips in egg and oil mix. Preheat the oven to 230C/gas 9. Melt coconut oil in base of oven dish and arrange chips in a layer. Roast for 25 minutes, turning halfway. Serve with Cod or Salmon or cheese and tomato omelette.

Vegemato Tempeh soup

10 plum tomatoes
Large handful of kale
Sea salt or pink himaylan salt
Black pepper
2 cloves of mashed garlic
2 spring onions, chopped
2 asparagus heads, chopped
2 stems of purple sprouting
Broccoli, chopped
1 stick of celery, sliced
6 cubes of Tempeh
Sprinkle of oregano
Sprinkle of parsley

Plunge 10 tomatoes into boiled water for 20 seconds. Transfer to a bowl of cold water. After 3 minutes remove and peel off skins. Blend in a liquidiser with chopped kale (remove stalks) and all seasoning with a cup of water. Put in a large saucepan with all vegetables and lightly fried garlic. Simmer for 15minutes adding cubed Tempeh for the last 5 minutes. If you're not vegan sprinkle. parmesan cheese on top before serving

Nutty egg salad

Half bulb of fennel, chopped.
Kohrabi, thinly sliced
Rocket and watercress leaves
Add dressing of choice
Handful of walnuts, chopped
2 hardboiled eggs and feta cheese

Put eggs in pan. Bring water to the boil. Boil eggs for 3 minutes. Put leaves on large plate and top with other ingredients, cubing the feta cheese. Remove shells from eggs. And chop for top layer of salad. Add beetroot for colour

Garlic Salad dressing

Dollop of sour cream
Chives, chopped
Mashed garlic, fried in butter
Shredded parsley
Pink Himalayan salt
Black pepper

Put all ingredients into a bowl and fold and stir. Cool garlic and add to mix. Spoon onto salad before serving.

RECIPES

Flax seed Salad dressing

Tbsp organic flax oil
Freshly squeezed lemon juice
Tsp balsamic vinegar
Sprinkle of chilli flakes or
Paprika

Put all ingredients into a bowl and stir before serving.

Mayonnaise

2 free range eggs, separated
250ml olive oil, cold pressed
1tsp Dijon mustard
1 tbsp fresh lemon juice
1 tsp white wine vinegar

Leave ingredients out so all are at room temperature. Blend egg yolks, mustard, lemon juice and white wine vinegar in a blender. Remove and slowly blend the olive oil with mixture. Add chopped dill and tarragon and serve with salad, artichokes and baked tuna or trout

Avocado and mint sauce

1 ripe avocado, sliced
1 tbsp fresh, chopped mint
100 ml sour cream
Salt and pepper
2 tsp fresh lime juice

Put avocado, sour cream and lime juice in a blender. Fold in chopped mint and seasoning and cover for an hour in the fridge before serving. Serve with Swiss chard, crayfish, thin slices of brie and vine ripened tomatoes.

Arty salad

Broad beans
Edam or Gouda cheese
Bok choi
Artichokes
Vine ripened tomatoes
Chopped oregano
Mackerel or sardines

Slice bok choi and arrange on a plate with all other vegetables and small strips of cheese. Grill fish for a few minutes and place on top of salad. Add dressing of choice.

Tarragon lemon summer squash soup

1 large yellow summer squash
2 green onions
1 tbspn butter
1 tbspn coconut oil
Fresh tarragon, chopped
1 garlic clove, parmesan cheese
Black pepper
Half cup plain yogurt
Lemon juice

RECIPES

Sauté the onion and squash in coconut oil and butter for 10 minutes. Add garlic for the last minute. Season with black pepper. Add tarragon and lemon juice and stir Cover and simmer for 15 minutes until squash is tender Add yogurt. Remove from heat and put into blender. Once blended, simmer for five more minutes. Sprinkle parmesan cheese on top before serving

Fruity pud

3 plums and 2 peaches, fresh
Half tsp each of nutmeg and cinnamon
Cardamom pods
Tblspn manuka honey
2 tblspns of fromage frais.
1 tbspn Ginger liqueur (optional)
1 cup berry herbal tea

Boil kettle and steep berry teabag for 5 minutes.
Wash and chop the fruit and stew it in berry tea.
Add cardamom pods, nutmeg and cinnamon.
Spoon in honey and stir. Add liqueur.
Serve after 5 minutes of stewing with fromage frais.

RELATIONSHIPS

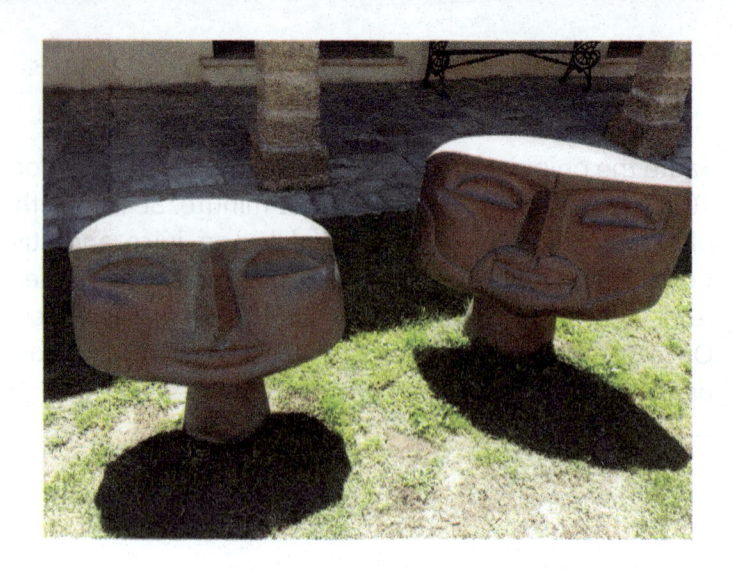

Your relationships with partners will have a direct affect on your mental, emotional and ultimately, physical health. When you first meet a man or woman there may be a chemical attraction, something that you just can't explain. It is intoxicating, but doesn't mean that it will be a stable, successful pairing.

The initial stages of a relationship involve setting up the rules or guidelines of what is acceptable to you. That may differ widely from person to person.

There will always be compromise in a relationship and although we hope that it will be drawn along with equanimity, one partner may be stronger or more assertive than the other. If you're an easy going, relaxed person who dislikes confrontation, you'll need to keep an eye on your boundaries so that your needs, opinions and wishes are not constantly overlooked.

A toxic relationship is one in which there is control and some form of verbal, mental, emotional or physical abuse. If you're dating or living with a man who subtly manipulates you into spending all your time with him, discouraging you when you make plans to see your family and friends, discuss it with him. If it continues, then leave.

Abuse can be veiled and subtle and aims to lower your self esteem. Your partner may initially seem warm and loving, and if you've been neglected and hurt you might finally feel that you've bonded with "the one". Do not tolerate abuse in any form from a partner.

Avoiding pain in life is rare and just not feasible. We all carry our experiences along with us as we mature and develop. MINDFULNESS and MEDITATION are essential life tools to observe what we allow ourselves to think and feel. Once we start to do that we become more self aware and conscious of our baggage or 'scripts' and stories that we tell ourselves. Our inner dialogue (which may be compounding negative beliefs about ourselves), or 'triggers' from past emotional experiences, may be carried into, and acted upon, in our current and future relationships.

Without constantly monitoring and feeling as if the relationship is under a microscope, notice if your partner makes derogatory comments about your weight, appearance, intellect and choices you make in your life. If this is not seen as positive or constructive you can decide to quietly, but firmly and clearly, challenge those comments.

Unhealthy relationships have an element of fear in them. Your partner may be making those comments because their sense of self worth is low and they fear you'll leave them.

Communication is key in your relationship and if there's a lot of common ground, mutual respect, patience and the ability to really listen, then solutions can be found.

Talk honestly about how you feel; wording sentences so that they're not aggressive, blaming or judgemental. Start by saying "I feel that.... ", which takes the onus off the sentence being directed at your partner and intimating that they are wrong or bad. Give them space to consider your emotions. Avoid yelling and becoming defensive when your partner retorts indignantly. Give them time to speak too and avoid interrupting. Communicating regularly can be awkward and uncomfortable but may mean that you can develop a loving, long term relationship based on mutual respect.

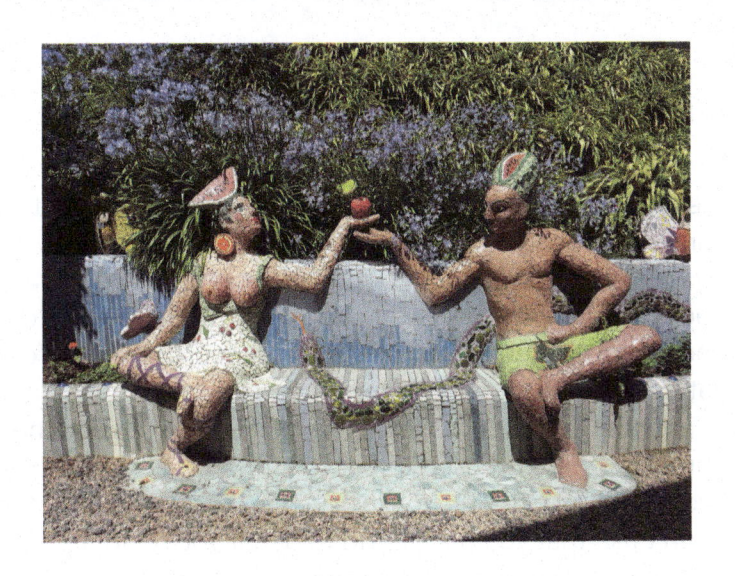

SEX

Love making, sex, intercourse are all words relating to a joining of bodies and will mean different things to different people. Some RELATIONSHIPS thrive on sex a few times a month and some every day. Finding a partner with a similar sex drive and expectations of how and how often will contribute to the smooth running of your relationship.

There will be times in your life when you just don't feel like it and your desire and libido drops. The CONTRACEPTIVE pill may contribute to this drop. After the birth of your baby you might be too exhausted. MENOPAUSE can make penetration uncomfortable. Discuss any issues with your partner regularly to ensure that frustration does not build and adversely affect your lives together.

Your body is not something to abuse and open up to people who only want to cause you pain and humiliation. Choose your partners and people you sleep with carefully. Share your body with those who will respect it, because all of our experiences leave a mental and emotional imprint.

If you are sleeping around, ask yourself why. It may be linked to a high sex drive or an addiction to sex, or boredom. Other times it may be related to a need for attention, affection and connection to someone.

These days SEX is seen as an initial part of the dating process where it's used to get to know the person. Trust your gut and initial response on a third or fourth date and don't feel that you have to go to bed if you're not ready. If you decide to, and you find that you're not compatible in bed, at least you find out early on. However, I've had relationships with men where the sex seemed a disaster the first time, then developed into something that was satisfying after tactful communication.

Sex will become a divine connection when there is mutual respect, knowledge and LOVE. It can still be physically pleasurable if those conditions are not there, but if you feel hollow, used and lonely after casual sex and one night stands, you aren't nurturing yourself.

Our society has become insatiable. These days, sex is woven into advertising and partners for casual sex can be found on apps. If you feel you want to experiment with multiple partners and are content not to have an emotional connection afterwards, then these are the days to do it. Your safety is paramount though, and if you are using apps and regularly sleeping with strangers, let a friend know where you are. Does it make you feel liberated to use apps? Is it two fingers up to your family and teachers? This is not a sanctimonious, judging chapter. You will do exactly what you want as the choice is yours and women have fought long and hard for equality and the right to experiment with multiple partners. Keep asking yourself how it feels.

Never judge a women if she confides in you about sex and has decided not to sleep with anyone until she is very sure it will be long term. Only you know how you feel about sex. As and when you make your decisions, ensure that you love yourself.

Most of us won't orgasm through VAGINAL penetration so if you've been with your partner for awhile you could mention the coital alignment technique (CAT). If your partner is patient and willing to let go of just thrusting until he climaxes, he could bring you to climax while he's inside you. Mention this to him and try it. Instead of thrusting, your man needs to lie on top of you with his pelvis higher than yours. By gently rocking in synchronicity your clitoris will be stimulated which means you may orgasm together with practise.

Sex changes over the decades but can still be enjoyed into your mature years.

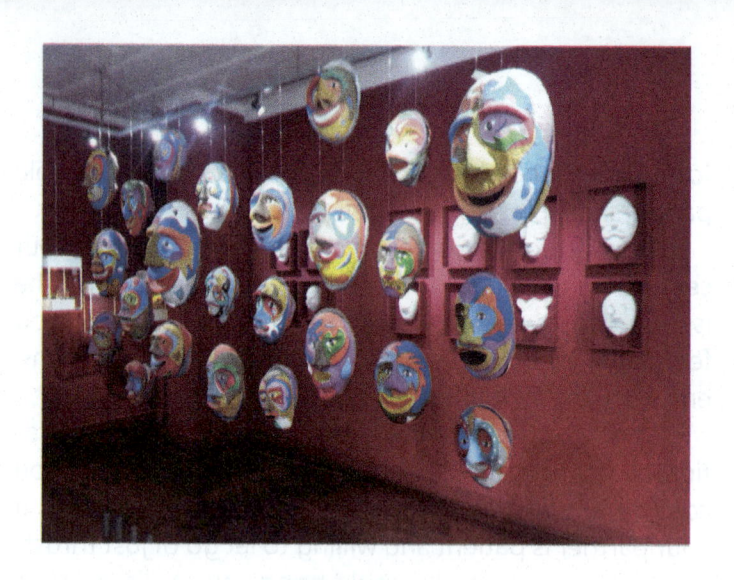

SKIN

Our skin absorbs around seventy percent of what we put on it. Skin helps in the regulation of body temperature. There are two main layers, the epidermis and dermis. Sweat and oil glands in the dermis, the lower layer, allow for sebum (oil) to be excreted from sebaceous glands and perspiration to be excreted from sweat glands.

Melanin is the pigment secreted by melanocytes in the skin. Sunlight darkens the skin due to melanin. There is a fatty substance in the skin which converts ultraviolet light from the sun to be converted to VITAMIN D. Along with the MINERALS calcium and phosphorus this is used to format and maintain bones in the body. It's now known that this direct sunlight positively impacts health. Find a balance where you get some sun for a short time (before or after the hours of midday) without sunscreen. Avoid burning from the sun. An SPF lotion should be 15 or 30. An SPF of 30 will give you 97% protection against UVB rays. Avoid using the waterproofed and highly

SKIN

chemical sunscreens as these can irritate the skin. Check the chapter on PRODUCTS for alternative sunscreen

The dermis is under the epidermis and is interlaced with collagen fibres. This spongy support weakens and thins as we mature. Hair roots and follicles, blood vessels, lymph vessels and sensory nerve endings are also found in the dermis.

Always use a cleanser if you wear makeup, so that you remove it before bed. Some people like to use a toner after cleansing, but if not, apply a moisturiser suitable for your age and skin type. Look on the back of products. Read ADDITIVES, CHEMICALS and TOXINS so that you attempt to reduce the pollutants in your daily life. Totally avoid products containing microbeads as these do not break down, so affect the Environment. Try not to grow up only focused on your own little world. There's the Earth to consider, along with your personal impact on it. Your weekly routine should include a gentle exfoliate and a mask for your skin type. This is something you can include in a DETOX day, where you switch off your social media and unhook from technology.

Acne is a skin condition defined as having blackheads, pustules, pimples and papules on the face or back. In its extreme form, the pus filled spots become inflamed and turn into cysts. It mostly affects teenagers before or during puberty when there are changes in the HORMONAL system. It can be hereditary and occur later in life too.

The sebaceous glands in the skin that produce sebum normally just keep the skin pliable and supple. The epidermis or top layer is constantly shedding dead skin cells so the skin is renewed as new cells come to the surface. It takes around a month for this turnover.

When HORMONES change and surge before puberty more sebum (oil) is produced and secreted. The pores or tiny openings on the skin become blocked with dead skin cells and sebum. This plug or blockage is what causes the acne pimple. Most of us get pimples at sometime.

The bacteria that live on the skin also block the pore, so the pimple becomes red, tender and swollen. If it is left untreated, it can worsen and turn into a cyst. It is important not to pop or break the cyst. Acne can leave scarring on the skin if particularly bad.

Acne can also affect self esteem and confidence leading to anxiety and depression. Avoid making rude comments or laughing at anyone with acne. People appreciate KINDNESS when they are dealing with challenges.

It's tempting to scrub and over cleanse the skin with astringent and harsh products. That can strip the skin of its natural PH acid mantle and may aggravate the acne. Use a gentle cleanser twice a day, particularly if you have been perspiring. Wash your hands before and after you've cleansed the skin. Keep your hair clean if it tends to get oily.

All skin conditions will benefit from taking a balanced OMEGA supplement. Avoid an excess of SUGAR, cakes, milk chocolate, ALCOHOL, junk food, white bread, pasta and white rice if you have acne. Limit dairy products, except plain, natural yogurt. You are what you eat, and what you take in does affect your skin. Read the chapter on JUICING and try it.

If you wear makeup ensure that it's noncomedogenic or nonacnegenic. Check the package. You can buy products from the pharmacy or chemist to treat acne. Some products will contain Azelaic acid which comes from rye, barley and wheat. It will slow sebum production and helps to eliminate bacteria. This is a helpful product for darker skins, as acne can leave dark patches called melasma. Keloids are scars that look firm, raised and rubbery and are more prominent due to collagen healing the site. They can occur in extreme cases of acne or damage to the skin. A keloid forms within scar tissue and can be uncomfortable. They are a lot more common in people of African, Asian and Latino descent. Cryotherapy is a treatment where extreme cold is applied to the keloid.

Salicylic acid is also used in acne products as it breaks down pimples and aids in slowing down the shedding of skin cells inside the oil glands. This lessens the redness and swelling. Another ingredient used is sulphur, which loosens blackheads and pustules and is antibacterial.

Retin A or retinol contains Tretinoin, an acid form of VITAMIN A which exfoliates or removes the top layer of epidermis. Some products will make the skin red for a day or two. Avoid sun if you have acne. Try to use sunscreens that don't have too many chemicals in them.

Acne is temporary. You may be advised to take antibiotics if it's severe. Always take an acidophilus probiotic for a month if you do have to take antibiotics, as these will restabilise the BOWEL.

There are alternatives and ESSENTIAL OILS are effective on a physical as well as an emotional level with acne. I blend twenty ml of base oil (almond or borage seed) then add two drops of Chamomile German or Roman, three drops of tea tree, one of eucalyptus and three of bergamot. Mix them and apply lightly over the face. You may think it counterproductive to apply oil but it does work. I also put a drop of eucalyptus on a cotton bud and roll it gently over a pustule or cyst. I have made a toner for clients containing a hundred ml of apple cider vinegar with ten drops of lavender ESSENTIAL OIL and ten drops of Geranium.

Try taking the HERBS Echinacea and Yellow dock root for pustular acne, psoriasis and wet eczema. Include GARLIC capsules as a supplement. Go online to www.lovelula.com for the product by Kimberly Sayer. Ultra light organic facial moisturizer has been designed for oily and acne prone skin. It contains zinc oxide and titanium oxide to give a high SPF to guard against sun damage and green tea and aloe vera to heal and soothe.

Our self esteem is linked to thoughts and emotional states and can change, based on our appearance and skin. If you develop the skin condition Rosacea later in life, you may need to research it for natural alternatives to keeping it under control, as it can be distressing. Initial symptoms down the centre of the face will include flushing and redness, small spidery looking blood vessels (telangiectasia) and spots which may be pustules. The skin may feel more sensitive and itch or burn and thicken with dry, rough patches. It's not known what exactly causes Rosacea, but there are theories regarding peptides, which are molecules within the skin.

Rosacea may worsen if you drink ALCOHOL, in particular red wine, hot drinks and caffeine, exposing your face to the sun for too long, and being in extreme temperatures, either too hot or cold or humidity. If you take corticosteroids, it can aggravate it. Other triggers include; spicy foods, MENOPAUSE, strenuous exercise, dairy products and stress.

When you have Rosacea there are a much higher number of demodex folliculorum on the skin. These

SKIN

are microscopic mites which sit on the human skin and don't normally cause problems, but in rosacea there is a theory that the skin reacts to bacteria from the mites' waste products (faeces). There is also speculation that helicobacter pylori bacteria (which causes ulcers in the stomach) may stimulate the production of bradykinin, which is a protein known to expand blood vessels.

As an aroma therapist, I have treated women with rosacea and made a blend of ESSENTIAL OILS with a base of 20 ml with an equal measure of carrot oil and jojoba. Jojoba is antibacterial and is close to our natural sebum. The most effective oils for reddened, irritated skin are styptic. You can blend night oil. I use three drops of Geranium, three of Cypress as these are effective for dilating blood capillaries, and three of German Chamomile, as this last oil is anti inflammatory and soothing. These nine drops are gently shaken in a glass bottle in the base oil, and then applied lightly over the face. Always store these oils in a dark, glass bottle. Women tend to use a cream during the day, so I advise them to put 1 drop of Eucalyptus into their daily moisturiser as this is antiseptic and cooling.

The skin condition Psoriasis is an autoimmune condition where the immune system attacks the body's cells. It is recognised by silvery scales and inflamed plaques on the face, scalp or joints. Exposure to the sun can help or special sun beds. Tar treatments are still offered. I blend three drops of Bergamot, three of tea tree, one of lavender in twenty ml of a jojoba and carrot base oil to apply to psoriasis.

Read the chapter on HERBS and ESSENTIAL OILS and see a nutritionist for advice on food allergies and intolerances if suffering with SKIN complaints and dermatitis and eczema.

SLEEP

For optimal health ensure that you get seven to nine hours sleep, when you can. Studies show that your physical and mental health will suffer if you are sleep deprived over a long period. It's now thought that to set your body clock, it's wise to go to bed and to get up at the same time every day. Levels of the HORMONE Cortisol will rise due to stress and sleeplessness, causing you to store fat around your belly.

If you're sleep deprived the hormone Ghrelin will increase by around 28%, so you'll feel hungrier than usual making lack of sleep a factor in obesity and weight gain. Sleepless nights may also lower Leptin levels, the hormone which reduces hunger pangs and tells your brain there's no need for more food.

In MENOPAUSE a drop in oestrogen affects sleep, causing women to wake in the night or to have trouble dropping off initially. Read the chapters on HERBS and ESSENTIAL OILS for natural remedies. Wear natural fibre clothes such as cotton, hemp or bamboo in bed, not synthetic. Read the chapter on HORMONES about Melatonin and order it online to try it for a few months. A small snack of carbohydrates can help relax you before bed so have an oat biscuit or a very small bowl of porridge (but not any other cereal). I occasionally take the HERB Valerian before bed too, if I'm feeling anxious or upset and something's on my mind.

In the hour before you go to bed turn off all electronic devices, including your Kindle. Electromagnetic fields can disrupt your thyroid gland which regulates metabolism and the pineal gland in your brain, which produces the sleep HORMONE Melatonin, and the 'feel good' one, serotonin. Take a break from your PC and iPad. If you're always on social media sites or are self employed (so dictate your own hours), and sometimes catch up late at night, this can be challenging. The blue light emitted from some devices will ensure the brain stays active. Bright light supresses melatonin, the sleep hormone, so for a beneficial night's sleep, ensure the room is very dark in whatever way you can, and allow yourself to start to switch off mentally.

Avoid exercise a couple of hours before bed and have a warm bath with a few drops of Lavender oil in a teaspoon of milk. Drink a cup of Chamomile tea or sleepy tea with lavender flower, limeflower, valerian root and lettuce. The tea company Pukka do an excellent one called night time. Try their range of wonderful teas.

If your bedroom is very warm it can impede sleep and have an impact on weight loss. Keep the temperature as low as 65 degrees Fahrenheit. This theory links into 'brown fat' which keeps your body warm by burning stored fat and regulating blood sugar.

Be aware of what you watch on TV if you want undisturbed sleep. Instead, invest in a relaxation or meditation CD or music you find relaxing and listen to it in the bath. Read a magazine or novel once in bed and feel that you need to let the day go, whatever's happened in it.

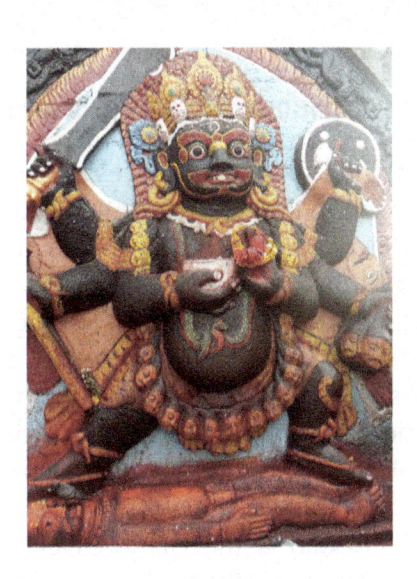

SUGAR

Diet coke and soda will poison your system. Treat yourself to one a week as a fix or give them up if you can. Most of us have some cake, chocolate, biscuits and ALCOHOL during the week, but try to limit it to an occasional treat, as it takes much longer than you think to burn off those calories in the gym. There are literally teaspoons of sugar in a glass of wine. Sugar is addictive.

Sugar is 'hidden' in processed and packaged food. Check the labels for sucralose (Splenda), neotame, acesulfame K, aspartame and saccharin. Avoid using these sweeteners. They fool your system into initially thinking it has had something sweet. When your brain realises it hasn't, it will want carbohydrates. Artificial sweeteners will also disrupt the microbiome or beneficial "good" bacteria and flora in your BOWEL. This microbiome in your gut is essential for optimal health. Sweeteners raise your insulin levels and blood sugar levels which could lead to weight gain and ill health.

Cereals, tinned soups and sauces in jars may contain an additional ten to fifteen teaspoons of addictive, teeth rotting, BOWEL destabilising sugar. Zero drinks and diet coke are one of the outrages of our times.

Our hospitals and dentists are seeing an unprecedented rise in tooth decay in children and adults due to sugary drinks. An unacceptable number of teenagers are obese and heading for a lifetime of self regulation due to type 2 Diabetes. An unnerving amount of people have limbs amputated from diabetes and excessive sugar consumption. Insulin is the HORMONE secreted from the pancreas that allows the body to use glucose. When you eat carbohydrates and they start to turn into sugar in the stomach, glucose in the blood stream stimulates the pancreas to release insulin. When you develop Type 2 diabetes the cells in your body cannot use glucose efficiently. This is known as insulin resistance as the pancreas will become unable to produce the correct amount of insulin.

Women do die from heart attacks. If you develop diabetes your risk of heart problems increases as blood vessels are damaged. Ensure you EXERCISE at least a few times a week.

Symptoms of diabetes include; excessive thirst, headaches, URINARY tract infections, vaginal dryness and loss of libido, fatigue and blurred vision. If you have a cut or wound, it will take longer to heal if you have diabetes.

Certain ethnic groups are at risk of type 2 diabetes. These include; Asians, African Americans, Native Americans and Hispanics. If someone in your family has diabetes you are more likely to develop it. If you had

SUGAR

gestational diabetes whilst pregnant, you have a higher risk of developing type 2 diabetes later.

Limit microwave dinners and eat more natural, non packaged food.

Avoid all artificial sweeteners (if you have to use a sweetener use Stevia, which is natural, sparingly). Read the chapter on XYLITOL. Avoid aspartame and start to gradually reduce the number of teaspoons of white sugar if you heap it into tea and coffee. It's not an exaggeration to say that sugar can be a killer.

Aspartame and artificial sweeteners are sweet tasting, but don't deliver the actual sugar your brain is expecting, so you head for the carbohydrates as your appetite is stimulated. Menthol toxicity is linked to aspartame due to the formaldehyde it converts into, which builds up in your system. Formaldehyde is a chemical preservative. Chewing gum contains sweeteners. Use tea tree or peppermint ESSENTIAL OILS in COCONUT oil as a mouthwash instead.

Dates and ripe bananas are an option if you're craving something sweet, so put them in your smoothies, desserts, porridge or just mash them up. Dates are a good source of fibre which slows the release of fruit sugar. Dates also contain the MINERALS calcium, IRON, magnesium, potassium and copper. Dried fruits are high in sugar and more challenging to digest. Buy apricots and dates that haven't been treated with the preservative sulphur dioxide as it is toxic. When fruits are dried the WATER is removed so wash them then soak them in filtered water for a few hours. Remove any pips or stones then put them in a blender with water. Use this sparingly as a spread or in porridge or smoothies.

I stew apples in cinnamon and a teaspoon of manuka honey, if I'm craving something sweet. Give this to your children as a snack and avoid taking them to places where sweets are on their eye level in shops and checkout counters. Other options are maple syrup and coconut sugar. Agave nectar is not a healthier option as it is higher in fructose than honey. Wean yourself off brown and white sugar and use half a teaspoon of organic honey or XYLITOL to cook with and to sweeten tea and coffee if you really need it.

Huge, greedy companies have figured out the ratios and magic proportions of fat and sugar to keep you hooked, fat and lethargic while they get richer and richer. When we eat or drink sweet things, our BRAINS release dopamine, which activates the brain's reward system. Even if you're skinny, avoid sweeteners. Will power, EXERCISE, being occupied and having encouraging people around you who know your goals, are what you will need to do to control the urges if you have been told you are obese. This can be even more challenging when you're premenstrual or going through MENOPAUSE.

Tests and research show that sugar is as addictive as recreational drugs. Hidden sugar in processed foods trigger neurons in your brain's pleasure centre and natural opiods and you can become addicted. Exercise and taking the MINERAL magnesium as a supplement will lower the craving for sugar. Sugar is toxic to your system and sets the scene for 'glucose intolerance', insulin resistance and diabetes. When there's too much sugar in your blood stream, your pancreas pumps more insulin into your system. If you become "insulin resistant" due to this you may eventually develop type 2 Diabetes. Once you have diabetes you either take tablets or self

SUGAR

inject and may end up with macular degeneration when your eyesight fails or in extreme cases, losing a limb. This is on the increase and our surgeons are under pressure to remove limbs and teeth owing to excess sugar in diets.

The 'good' bacteria or flora in our BOWEL and gut contribute hugely to our overall health and wellbeing and sugar disrupts this balance. Candida Albicans, a yeast that can affect your health badly once it has become lodged in your system, feeds off sugar, as does cancer. Taking the contraceptive pill over a long period and excessive use of antibiotics can lead to Candida.

The only sugar you should have in your diet is raw, organic honey or Manuka honey. There are other sweet alternatives, so read the chapter XYLITOL so you can start to use them. Use honey sparingly (I have a third of a teaspoon in my green tea) and don't kid yourself that Agave syrup is natural and beneficial. It's not. It actually has more fructose in it than sugar, and fructose is the big baddy. Fructose turns into "free fatty acids" (the damaging form of cholesterol) and triglycerides, which will ultimately turn into fat on you. Fructose breaks down into a harmful waste product called uric acid which increases your blood pressure. Your liver works hard as it's the sorting and clearing house dealing with anything that comes into your body and it struggles to metabolize fructose. Check all labels for High Fructose Corn Syrup and avoid it like the bubonic plague.

The hormone leptin suppresses appetite but fructose interferes with this message in your body which means you're likely to have some more. Sugar also affects the efficiency of the brain neurotransmitter dopamine.

Sugar molecules bond to protein molecules leading to the formation of cross linked proteins. This is known as glycosylation and leads to your body aging instead of creating new cells and tissue.

Your HORMONAL system is disrupted by constantly monitoring sugar intake and blood sugar levels.

Stop buying 'low fat' or 'light' foods as these are generally loaded with sugar or sweeteners, and it's the body's storage of this that actually contributes to making you fat. There are three kinds of sugar; glucose, sucrose and fructose. Fructose is found naturally in whole fruit, which in moderation should be part of your diet as it contains antioxidants, VITAMINS and fibre. Some fibre is essential when on a weight loss program and for optimal BOWEL health.

If you're juicing, focus more on VEGETABLES but limit the fruit. Fructose is slightly lower on the Glycemic index compared to sucrose and glucose but metabolically, it's a disaster when processed. It's a lie that fruit juice should be one of your 'five a day'. Fruit juice is a fibreless sugar bomb so drink it sparingly, watered down, as a treat. If you're trying to lose weight and for a few months are increasing protein and decreasing carbohydrates, then only have blueberries and the occasional apple. Raisins and sultanas are also inordinately high in sugar, so they're not an ideal snack. Have an apple or pear instead. Once you have stabilised your blood sugar level you can have a little more fruit, but VEGETABLES should make up most of your weekly diet.

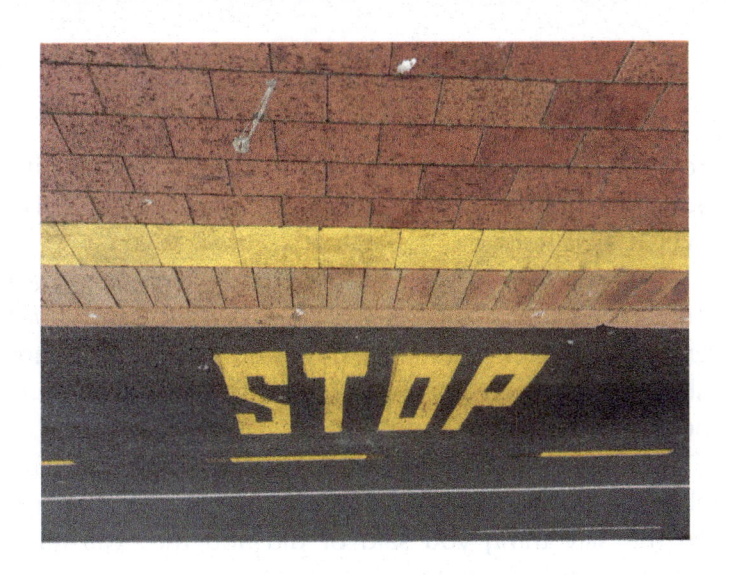

THOUGHTS

If you think you can, you're right and if you think you can't you're right. This is a simple line to teach your children and to let them know that whatever they think about constantly may manifest in their lives and actually materialise. What we allow ourselves to think about from the moment we wake up, until we fall into dreamy sleep directly influences our everyday experience of the world. Is that a snake on the path or a coiled rope? Are you sure? Milton wrote "The mind is its own place, and in itself can make a heaven of Hell, a Hell of Heaven".

If you live a life where you expect external influences and people to make you happy, you may become disillusioned and disappointed. If you're depending on something or someone that you can't control to keep you happy, you may find yourself in a world of pain. What we think about leads to emotions. Be watchful of your thoughts and the emotions they lead into as constant negativity will eventually manifest as physical ill health.

You must create your contentment and satisfaction with your thoughts and expectations. Practising GRATITUDE every day is helpful.

We go through our days experiencing what we perceive as "pain" and "pleasure". Experiences, however embarrassing or traumatic they seem at the time, are all temporary and transient. Ensure your self esteem is healthy, but take yourself lightly.

It's none of your business what other people think about you. Most of the time people are not dwelling on the silly thing you said or did and they will have forgotten about it before you.

However, think before you speak or gossip about other people as this is poisonous behaviour. Do not get involved in any kind of malicious gossip on social media or life. Think about how it would feel to be in a situation where you felt isolated and ridiculed. Think about how KINDNESS ripples out when you experience it, and use that whenever you can, even when a situation or a person seems difficult.

TOXIC

It's now known that food dyes, colouring and additives affect some children's behaviour, contributing to them becoming hyper active and unruly. Look on the supermarket packages and boxes. The labels state 'artificial' flavour so we actually have no idea what chemicals we're ingesting along with our food. Ultimately, it would be wise to only cook whole, fresh food and not ready meals, although these have improved and some companies have decreased the amount of fat and sugar in theirs.

Start checking the amount of anti nutrients which are just loaded calories. I occasionally buy tomato sauces in jars, but lately have been putting fresh vine ripened tomatoes in my blender with garlic and Cajun pepper, and using that instead. Anything in a tin or jar is likely to have added SUGAR in it. If you want to live a longer, healthier, pain free life then eliminate or dramatically decrease the amount of junk food you buy and consume mindlessly in front of the TV.

These are some of the additives in food that are best avoided. Nitrates and Nitrites are detrimental to health. Sodium Nitrite is the synthetic preservative in meat that makes it look pink. If the meat is heated the nitrites turn into nitrosamines which have been linked to causing cancer of the bladder, pancreas, stomach and colon. Avoid beef burgers, sausages and hot dogs in excess and don't feed them to your children. Buy grass fed, organically reared meat if you eat it, but try to increase the amount of vegetables, pulses and beans you eat, because you may be swallowing antibiotics and growth hormones along with your poultry and meat. Get creative with vegetables in RECIPES.

Nitrates by themselves are actually present in some vegetables. They only become toxic in meat products and suspected carcinogens, when heated and combined with amines to become nitrosamines. It's the nitrosamines that increase your chances of degenerative disease.

Butylated Hydroxyanisole (BHA) is a suspected carcinogen. It's found in a lot of processed food such as popcorn, crisps, chips and some cereals and could be linked to allergic reactions, hyper activity and mood changes, as it affects the neurological part of the brain. Microwave popcorn bags are toxic. The bags containing the popcorn can have a chemical known as perfluoroctanoic (PFOA) acid in them. Studies on PFOA have linked it to liver, bladder, testicular, kidney and pancreatic cancer. The actual popcorn might be made with soybean which is genetically modified and may affect your long term health. Some crisps contain artificial colours, trans fats and preservatives. Crisps are fried at high temperatures which create a substance known as acrylamide, a known carcinogen, which is also found in cigarettes. Keep an eye on what the men in your life are snacking on.

Butylated Hydroxytoluene (BHT) is a chemical added to food which has caused thyroid hormonal changes in animal tests. The thyroid gland in your neck regulates metabolism and is linked to the Hypothalamus in your BRAIN.

The chemical Potassium Bromate is added to flour to make bread, buns and rolls more pliable but also unbalances the finely tuned thyroid and hormonal system while contributing to digestive discomfort and kidney damage. Some countries have banned Potassium Bromate as an additive. White flour is bleached with chlorine. Brown bread might just have colour and SUGAR added to it. A sandwich is a staple snack in a lot of countries, so some people consume bread every day and for most it's not a problem, but try more salads in the summer and homemade soups in the winter.

Propyl Paraben is found in food dyes, muffins, tortillas and has an oestrogenic effect so could be a factor in speeding up the growth of breast cancer cells, affecting testosterone levels and sperm count in men. Think twice before spending your hard earned cash on packaged and processed food with these substances in them. Check the labels before you buy them.

Sulphur Dioxide is a sulphite and is in the air we breathe. High Sulphur Dioxide levels can be harmful if we live and work in a large, polluted city where coal and fuel are burned. It's increased in the last hundred years as manufacturers use it as a cheap, effective preservative. In a long list of foodstuff sulphur dioxide is known as E220 in Europe. Sulfites are also used in preserved, processed meat such as sausages, beers, potatoes, some dried fruit and desiccated coconut. A small number of people are adversely affected by sulphur dioxide and some believe it has contributed to the rise in Asthma cases. If you are asthmatic you may want to avoid white wine, in particular sweet Bordeaux, Loire and German wines. If you drink a lot of white wine you'll be ingesting more sulphites than most.

Monosodium Glutamate is a flavour enhancer (Doritos and pot noodles). It's been linked to heart palpitations, numbness, headaches, nausea, fatty liver, high insulin, neurological imbalances and fibromyalgia. You can check packets of food for this so that you can avoid it. It comes in various disguises. Here's a list of them; E621, E620, monopotassium, glutamate, monoammonium glutamate(E624), calcium glutamate(E623), Yeast extract, natrium glutamate, hydrolized protein, calcium caseinate, sodium caseinate, autolyzed yeast, textured protein. Limit maltodextrin and malt extract in your diet.

Glutamic acid is actually a neurotransmitter used by the brain, nervous system and pancreas.

Many people have started to work on allotments or grow their own vegetables and fruit in pots in their back gardens or on balconies as you'll avoid plastic packaging, GENETICALLY MODIFIED food and chemical pesticides.

URINARY

You may have a urinary tract infection if you have a burning sensation when urinating, pain in your abdomen and a fever. Urethritis is inflammation of the urethra, the tube from the bladder.

Cystitis is a urinary tract infection caused by bacteria and inflammation of the lining of the bladder. You will feel an urgent need to urinate but there won't be much urine. If it's extreme, there may be blood in your urine. You may have stomach pain and a fever. If there is a lot of blood, go to your doctor as this can be indicative of bladder or kidney disease.

Stress, excessive sex, bruising during penetrative intercourse, antibiotics, excessive sugar and the CONTRACEPTIVE pill can cause cystitis. Go to your doctor so that you can start and finish a course of antibiotics. Drink sugar free cranberry juice to normalise the PH level. It's essential to take a probiotic with acidophilus after antibiotics. Eat plain, natural yogurt. Read the chapter on ESSENTIAL OILS to ease the discomfort of urinary tract infections. Make sure you urinate straight after sex to flush out any bacteria that may be lurking. If you can't get to the doctor quickly, drink a quarter of a tablespoon of baking soda (bicarbonate) in a large glass of water. This is thought of as a cure all for many things.

A TO Z MINI-GUIDE TO WOMEN'S HEALTH

Always wipe front to back after a bowel movement. Use mild soap, not heavily perfumed or scented bubble baths. Check the labels for chemicals so that products you regularly use are as natural as possible.

US

We are all interdependent and reliant on each other, as we make our way through our own little personal worlds, lives and routines. It's so easy to forget that the small choices and decisions we make on an hourly basis affect the globe, the Earth and all who live here. What happens in the clearing of a rain forest in South America to plant palm oil, will ultimately affect us all but we shrug our shoulders and wonder what we could possibly do to reduce the impact of this destruction.

Most of us won't join Greenpeace and tie ourselves to trees, but it's time to make measured, conscious decisions and plans to ensure that there is a planet that's sustainable for future generations. Children could be educated from a young age about what's really important, not designer brands or the latest smartphone, but allotments and recycling. Join Friends of the Earth and other organisations and support them with small donations and by signing petitions. It seems unthinkable that by the time your young children are middle aged there won't be any polar bears or elephants or tigers left on Earth.

Small gestures such as using green products, like Ecover, instead of bleach and chemicals when we clean, contribute to the stability of our aquatic life and water quality. Some countries are way ahead of others in regard to banning bleach, using solar panels, eliminating plastic bags from supermarkets, composting food waste, utilising a water holder for rain in the garden and insisting that their governments ban pesticides (neonicotinoids) that wreak havoc on our bee colonies and their ability to pollinate our food. Einstein stated that if the bees die off we will struggle to produce plants. Many species of bees have already been decimated.

Food will become extortionately priced, as we navigate through the growing issue of millions of people going hungry in certain parts of the world, already ravaged by global warming and changing weather patterns. We already use vast tracts of land for cattle and livestock and have depleted thousands of acres of soil by abandoning crop rotation and sustainable methods.

Become proactive. Sign petitions online and become responsible and accountable as an individual. We all use electricity, gas and most of us drive cars and have a long haul flight once a year, but we can lighten our carbon footprint and inform our governments of our disgust and incredulity at their short term policies. No man is an island, but sometimes it takes a personal affront for us as individuals to finally contemplate the end game and the Earth dying. Sound dramatic? If we don't take action as a collective, it could be chaos sooner than we imagined.

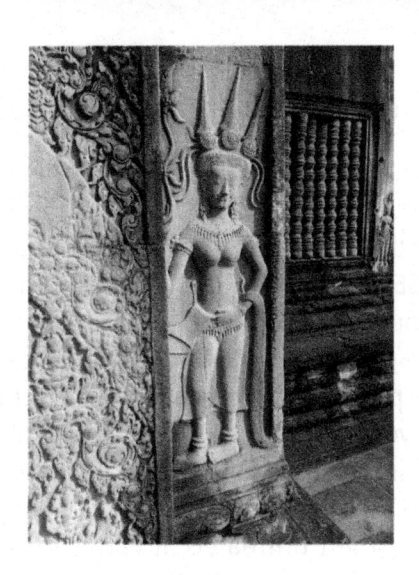

UTERUS

The womb or uterus is situated in the pelvic cavity between the bladder and the rectum (end of the bowels). It is supported by ligaments and muscles. As an important aspect of a woman, it's the place an embryo beds in and develops into a baby. It is hollow, muscular and pear shaped.

The fundus is the dome shaped part of the uterus which is just above the openings of the uterine (fallopian) tubes. The low, narrow part of the uterus leads to the cervix, the connection which protrudes into the VAGINA or birth canal. The uterine tubes extend from the sides of the uterus. At the ends of the two tubes are finger like projections which are close to the ovaries. The uterine tubes move a fertilized egg or ovum down into the uterus to begin its forty week development. During labour, the uterus contracts, the cervix relaxes and opens to allow the birth.

Prolapse or dropping occurs when the uterus sags towards the vagina. This can occur when levels of the female HORMONE oestrogen decline during or after MENOPAUSE, as this HORMONE maintains strength in the pelvic muscles.

Difficult pregnancies and childbirth can also contribute to a prolapsed uterus. If you have the following symptoms you may be at risk; vaginal bleeding, discomfort during sexual intercourse, increased discharge, constipation, bladder infections and pulling sensations in the pelvis. If left untreated, it can lead to bowel and bladder problems. If you suffer from heavy bleeding (menometrorhagia) between periods, go and see your doctor.

Uterine prolapse is diagnosed by inserting a device inside the vagina to see if the uterus is evident. The pelvic ligaments can be secured and reattached. If it's not severe you may be able to prevent it from deteriorating by practising Pilates, Kegel exercises which strengthen the pelvic floor or taking HRT (hormone replacement therapy). Read the chapter on MENOPAUSE for more information on HRT. Pessaries can be inserted up into the vagina as support. Avoid lifting heavy weights and lose weight if you've been told you are obese.

Surgery in the form of hysterectomy, where the uterus is removed either through the vagina or an incision in the abdomen, may be offered. This surgery is not as common as it once was, and unless there is widespread disease, can be avoided. Hysterectomy kick starts menopause and can lead in some cases to loss of well being and sexuality, where there is a decline in libido. The VAGINA can become dry and narrow and intercourse uncomfortable, if there is obstructive scar

UTERUS

tissue after a hysterectomy. Research has shown that if you do have a hysterectomy you may have to take hormone replacement therapy (HRT). When the primarily male hormone testosterone decreases in women, energy and confidence can drop.

Fibroids (fleshy cysts) in the reproductive area are fairly common. They may have developed because of HORMONAL imbalances and the over production of oestrogen. Read the chapter on MENOPAUSE for more information about oestrogen. The CONTRACEPTIVE pill can contribute to fibroids. Fibroids are normally benign or non cancerous. They can cause heavy, painful periods. If you have them, penetrative sex can be uncomfortable and your FERTILITY may be impaired.

Endometriosis can also adversely affect your chances of conceiving naturally. When you have this debilitating condition the cells lining the uterus are also found in other parts of the body. Every month our HORMONES prepare the uterus for an anticipated pregnancy. When this doesn't take place we have a release of the build up on the walls of the uterus. This is our monthly cycle or period. Our cycles are generally twenty eight days long. Every month the rogue cells that have found their way into other parts of the body, will act as if they are in the uterus, and will start to bleed. If you have very heavy, painful periods ask to be tested for this condition. If this is left and not treated it can affect your URINARY system and FERTILITY.

A gynaecological laparoscopy is a surgical procedure where the reproductive system can be examined. If there are symptoms mentioned in this chapter and in the one about OVARIES (ovarian cysts) you may be offered ultra sound or a laparoscopy. An opening is made in the abdomen so that a surgeon can investigate and take a biopsy if necessary. A biopsy is a small sample of tissue taken from the body which can be checked for cancer and other conditions. Endometriosis may be diagnosed after a laparoscopy. This surgical procedure can also be used to remove infection or previous scar tissue and to perform sterilisation, where the fallopian tubes are closed off to prevent further unwanted pregnancies. In some cases, where cancer is evident, an oophorectomy or removal of the ovaries will be performed.

Your uterus is a sacred space, not just an organ for a developing foetus. The uterus produces prostaglandins which help to regulate your immune system into old age. The prostaglandin, prostacylin, inhibits blood clotting, so helps prevent heart disease.

The body is constantly sending messages through cells, nerves and HORMONES. If you opt for a hysterectomy but have your ovaries left intact, your ovaries may not function as well as they did due to the connective aspect of your reproductive system. The incidence of cardiovascular and heart disease, osteoarthritis and depression may increase after hysterectomy. This makes a healthy diet, regular EXERCISE and MEDITATION of the utmost importance to offset this.

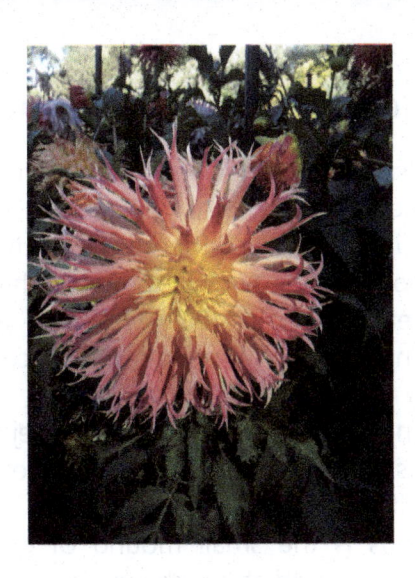

VAGINA

The vagina is a fibro muscular tube that connects to the cervix and reproductive system. The cervix is the neck of the UTERUS and connects the uterus to the vagina. The vagina's back wall is around nine centimetres long, but shape and size vary. The length of it can range from six to twelve centimetres and the width, between two or three centimetres. After having a baby the size may change. Just above the vaginal opening there is a small hole called the urethra which we urinate from.

The hymen is a thin layer of mucous membrane over the opening of the vagina, which can be broken during childhood from gymnastics, horse riding and vigorous activities or later, from intercourse. It does heal if torn and just becomes more flexible.

External genitalia or vulva are; the labia majora, two large folds of skin and fibrous tissue outside the vagina. Inside there are also two smaller folds of skin or inner lips known as labia minora which contain sebaceous or oil glands. These glands secrete sebum or oil which lubricate the vagina. These areas vary in size and appearance in women and there is no such thing as an ugly or abnormal one. Surgery on labias has increased in recent years to make this area more aesthetically pleasing. Why bother? We need to embrace our unique individuality.

The Skene glands swell and squirt or ejaculate fluid during arousal. So, it's not just men who ejaculate, but don't worry if you don't.

The clitoris is the small mound of erectile tissue with a protective hood above the vagina which contains numerous nerve endings, making it highly sensitive. It becomes erect, along with the labia, when stimulated and when gently circled or massaged during foreplay, sex or masturbation. This can lead to orgasm. Ask your partner for "butterfly fingers" around this area initially, so it is soft and gradual.

Your vaginal walls and uterus contract during orgasm. It's pleasant, enjoyable and relaxing to masturbate, so find out what brings you to orgasm, so that you can let a partner know. It relieves stress and can help you sleep. Try contracting the vagina just before you climax to increase the waves. Google the TED talk by Dr Jenn about sex and MINDFULNESS. Use a natural lubricant and your fingertips when masturbating. Lubrication can be very helpful if you're going through the MENOPAUSE as due to lowering of oestrogen the vaginal PH can change and the area may become thinner and dry even if you are aroused.

Stress can initiate a drop in Oestrogen, so less blood flows to the vagina, causing dryness. Your natural lubrication can lessen during Menopause.

VAGINA

Men who take their time with foreplay reap the benefits. Encourage lovers to spend at least fifteen minutes turning you on, as the vagina needs to be lubricated thoroughly before penetration. If you start a RELATIONSHIP with a man who has no knowledge of the significance or importance of gently stroking and teasing your clitoris, you can masturbate in front of him or guide his hand making encouraging comments and noises.

Cunnilingus is the act during which a man uses his tongue or lips on the clitoris and vagina area. The perineum is the area between the anus and vagina and also contains many nerve endings, making it an erogenous (sexually exciting) area for some people.

Women who have regular penetrative sex have healthier vaginas. Use it or lose it! For most women clitoral stimulation is the only way they orgasm. Less than a third of women orgasm from penile penetration.

The G spot is an area on the front of the vaginal wall and is linked to pleasure when stimulated.

We need to maintain a healthy PH balance in the vagina (PH is a scale of one to 14 indicating an acidic or alkaline state). Too much sugar, not enough rest or sleep or relaxation can lead to imbalance. If you take the CONTRACEPTIVE pill, wear tight nylon or synthetic pants and tights you may upset the delicate balance and PH of the vagina.

If you're exhausted and have discomfort or unusual, heavy discharge from the vagina, cut out SUGAR and go to a naturopath to be tested for candida. This is a fungal overgrowth that can occur in the digestive system and vagina. In the vagina it can cause thrush, which may be irritating when you urinate. You can spot it by a white discharge which looks like cottage cheese. It will be itchy and uncomfortable. If you go to your doctors you may be given antifungal pessaries to insert up the vagina. If you have candida, taking the HERB Pau d'arco and caprylic acid with acidophilus, which is a probiotic, will help in bringing your system back towards normality. Candida loves SUGAR and ALCOHOL so try not to feed it, as it will cause more than just thrush in the long term if it takes hold through your digestive system. Eat plain, natural yogurt, and take acidophilus supplements every time you have to take antibiotics to rebalance the healthy flora or bacteria in your system. Avoid antibiotics if you can.

Relactagel is a vaginal product that can be used in the vagina to help bring the PH and healthy bacteria back to optimal levels. If you've had thrush, tell your partner to go to the doctor too, as you may pass it between you. There is now a single dose anti fungal tablet you can take. Put five drops of Geranium and five of Tea tree ESSENTIAL oils in a warm bath too, as these are anti fungal. Take half a teaspoon a day of colloidal silver which will be available in a health food shop. This helps to eradicate bacterial and fungal infections in your body.

A fishy smell and frothy or thin discharge might be a sign that you have Gardnerella vaginalis. This is not something that you pass onto a partner, it happens due to stress or taking the pill. Rebalance the PH of the vagina by using a douche with a third of vinegar to two thirds of spring water.

Trichomoniasis is an infection that causes a very stinky, greenish yellow discharge. You'll need to give a sample of this to confirm it, and then take antibiotics.

It can be passed to a partner so you'll need to let them know, so they can be treated too.

During pregnancy it will be beneficial to massage the perineum with vegetable oil such as sweet almond to keep it pliable and flexible as it will be less likely to tear.

An episiotomy is a small cut made in the skin between the anus and vagina. It's a procedure that's used during childbirth to open the vagina if the baby seems distressed.

Your vagina may be a little wider after childbirth. During sex close your legs and contract upwards so it feels a little tighter for your partner. Accept the change as a natural part of parenthood.

Take up kegel exercises and Pilates after the birth to tone the pelvic floor.

Vaginal tension or vaginismus is a condition where the pelvic floor muscles involuntarily contract. Using tampons and having penetrative sex becomes difficult or impossible if you suffer with it. This can be due to physical reasons such as previous surgery, infection or irritated nerve endings. It can also be psychological and linked to earlier uncomfortable or painful sexual experiences. Anxiety is common with vaginismus, so counselling could be helpful. Physical treatments include inserting plastic tubes into the vagina which increase in size. MEDITATION and breathing techniques are always helpful in combating extreme stress and tension.

Every few years, or more if you're advised, it's essential that you go to your doctors for a pap smear test. The results can be abnormal occasionally, which doesn't mean it's life threatening. A pap smear helps to check if there are any cell changes that could turn into cervical cancer, but it is not one hundred percent effective in confirming this. The test checks for warts or Human papilloma virus (HPV). Over half of us carry the virus. There are over fifty two strains of HPV, but only two strains are linked to cervical cancer, so if you do have genital warts at some time from unprotected sex, it doesn't necessarily mean you will suffer from cervical cancer. If you have warts they will look like small lumps around the genital area. When you go to a nurse for a pap smear, a swab of cells is taken from the cervix by inserting a tube into the vagina. It should be painless, but try to relax internally and focus on breathing smoothly and fully the first time you go.

The Brazilian and Hollywood are names given to waxing the bikini pubic area. These are extreme so think twice, as it's lower maintenance and less painful to just wax the area outside of your actual, fabric bikini. You can carefully trim your pubic hairs with scissors or an epilady attachment for them. The pubic hair is taken out from the roots with warm wax when you go to a beautician for a bikini wax. I use tea tree ESSENTIAL OIL in aloe vera gel on the waxed area for a few days. If you notice lumps, spots and pustules you probably have an ingrown hair, which is common after waxing. These can become larger and infected, turning into boils, so keep checking the area. Use a light exfoliating scrub a week after the bikini wax, and do that gently once a week.

Your vagina is sacred space and through the ages has been revered and likened to a rose bud. Look after it well and be mindful of who you want to share it with. It will change as you mature, and if you have children, so just accept it as it is.

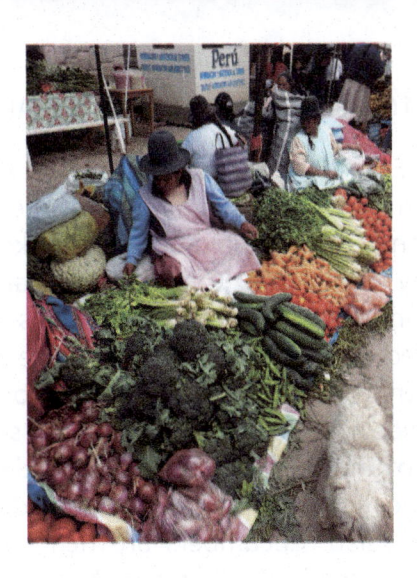

VEGETABLES

Vegetables should make up at least a third of your daily food intake and when used in soups, stews and curries can be delicious and nutritious. Get creative with them with herbs, spices and cheese and try different combinations with soups, as they give you a wide range of VITAMINS and MINERALS to prevent disease.

Munch on raw courgettes, peppers and celery for a crunchy snack. Dip them in guacamole or a small portion of humus. My latest soup has sweet potato, onions, garlic, Cajun spice with coconut milk and ementhal cheese which has been blended and simmered with chopped leeks and peas, popped in before serving. Parsley and celery contain a compound called apigenin which may be helpful in blocking blood vessel forming which feed cancer tumours in the BREAST. Research is ongoing (cancer research by Salman Hyder) but could help shrink tumours in breast tissue. If you are traversing

MENOPAUSE and are taking progestin in HRT, include parsley, celery and NUTS in your weekly diet.

I've recently grown Kohlrabi, which looks like a white turnip, in my tiny garden. Kohlrabi has an abundance of vitamins C and B6, folate and potassium as well as fibre. I like it grated on salads with goat's cheese and parsley.

I also enjoy grated turnip, golden beetroot and chopped sweetheart cabbage on a salad so there's an abundance of unusual flavours, textures and crunchiness. Red cabbage and the purple lettuce radicchio bring colour to a salad. Cucumbers are rich in silicon and sulphur that benefit the kidneys. The silica in them strengthens your nails and hair. I like to add some pine nuts or hazlenuts on top of the salad too. Every Christmas my mum cooks red cabbage with apples to enjoy with the sprouts. Roasted vegetables are enhanced with sprigs of rosemary and thyme. Turnip is nourishing and filling in a soup with leeks and a small amount of cream or crème fraiche.

If you're cooking these dishes and some of the family or your friends enjoy bacon, fry some up and add to their dish at the last minute. You could also add vegetarian sausages. Experiment with different combinations of HERBS and cheeses with your vegetables. You can grow pots of HERBS, fruit and vegetables, even if you only have a tiny space on a balcony or garden.

If you're on a high protein, low carbohydrate diet for a month avoid parsnips, potatoes, corn and lentils as these are more starchy, then gradually reintroduce them. Only have white potatoes as an occasional treat. (I have fish and chips once a year). Don't buy wilted, old vegetables and do keep them in the fridge.

VEGETABLES

Chicory contains fructo polysaccharides inulin and FOS. These are prebiotics which are essential for feeding the healthy bacteria in the BOWEL or gut. Your immune function and mental health depend on this area. As FOS and inulin are soluable types of fiber, they are indigestible so reach the large intestine, preventing constipation. They also aid in the removal of cholesterol through the BOWEL, balance blood sugar levels as they make you feel full, and are naturally sweet.

Mash up your cooked sweet potato with some butter, a shake of paprika and spoonful of mascarpone. If you're going through MENOPAUSE ensure you include celery and parsley in your diet once a week. Celery contains VITAMIN K for blood clotting and bones, iodine, the MINERAL that aids in making the HORMONES in the thyroid gland for metabolism and the minerals potassium and sodium. Celery is a natural diuretic and anti-inflammatory.

Asparagus contains high levels of folic acid the B vitamin so eat it if you're thinking about conceiving a child. Broccoli is a good source of phosphorus and calcium so excellent for your skeleton.

I trim Kale to take out the central stalk and recently cooked it with tomatoes, garlic, oregano, onion, carrots and mascarpone cheese. Kale is incredibly good for you and has more VITAMIN C than an orange. It also contains lots of vitamin A and K and the B- complex vitamins. Try Cavolo nero with deep, dark green-black leaves to get IRON from your vegetables.

The humble little green pea is anti-inflammatory and a nutrient powerhouse containing folate, VITAMINS K, D, A and C and the MINERALS manganese, calcium, copper, IRON and ZINC. Peas also contain the polyphenol, coumestrol, said to help reduce the chances of stomach cancer. You will need a willow wigwam or wooden supports to grow peas up in your garden as they climb. They are prolific and I always enjoy sitting in the garden shelling them in the summer.

I chop fennel into slivers then warm it with garlic in a pan with butter and a little water, then put it on salads with grated cheddar and a few walnuts or into homemade tomato soup. Romanesco cauliflowers are green with little pointy tops and are a stunning colour and tasty.

Squash is actually a fruit and is wonderful roasted with garlic or in a curry with spinach. There are many varieties of squash now. Spinach gives you energy, is rich in IRON, VITAMINS A and K and helps the body to absorb calcium. I am currently enjoying my veggie boxes from Abel and Cole.

Studies show that reducing starchy carbohydrates such as white rice, bread, white potatoes and pasta and increasing vegetable uptake decreases your risk of heart disease, stroke, cancer and diabetes and alkalises your body, as acidic systems are ripe for degenerative disease. You'll lose weight too. If you eat a lot of meat and sugary foods washed down with copious amounts of alcohol you'll have an acidic body. Bacteria, viruses and fungus thrive in an acidic body and if left unchecked, can cause fatigue and ill health.

Nutrient rich vegetables also contain fibre for BOWEL health. The B vitamins niacin, riboflavin, folate, B6 and B12 are essential for energy. Vegetables have an abundant amount of the anti oxidants VITAMINS A, C, E and K needed to prevent ageing and chronic disease by counteracting free radical damage in your cells.

VEGETABLES

In recent research VITAMIN D (take as D3, not D2 if you are tested as low and need a supplement) has been shown as an effective and important counter against degenerative disease. Taken as part of a nutrition plan, include K2 and magnesium for the body to use it optimally. It's now commonly believed to be effective against flu as it will destroy bacteria and viruses, prevent heart disease, autoimmune dysfunction (multiple sclerosis), lung disease, bladder and colon cancer and Alzheimers. Evidence now suggests vitamin D boosts your immune response, has an effect on nerves in brain tissue and assists in the repair of DNA. A moderate amount of sunlight is the cheapest, most effective way to ensure you stay topped up with vitamin D. Vitamin K or phylloquinone is fat soluble and is essential for the formation of prothrombin, one of the compounds needed for your blood to clot, so that you don't bleed to death in the event of an accident.

The best food sources are leafy green vegetables. In the summer, use different coloured vegetables. Try bok choi, which is rich in vitamin C, as a base and add chopped raw fennel or kohlrabi, plum tomatoes, artichokes and small spiced beetroot with goat's cheese. Watercress is top of the list in 'goodies' so include it in your salads along with other bitter tasting foods. Vegetables like artichokes, chicory and radicchio are bitter so are helpful for cleansing the liver, the sorting and clearing house in our systems. The exciting combinations are endless. Make your own dressing, particularly if you're on a weight loss plan, as shop bought dressings can contain a lot of fat, SUGAR, additives and extra calories. A good base for a healthy dressing is organic flax seed oil, the most balanced oil in regard to essential OMEGA oils with balsamic vinegar and fresh lemon or lime juice with ginger or paprika or lightly fried, crushed garlic. Shred and tear basil, coriander or parsley into your dressings. Buy good quality cold pressed oils and don't heat them as they change into damaging forms that your body can't use and so actually damage cells.

Fry occasionally with butter, lard or coconut oil. Avocados and tomatoes are technically fruits. Avocado is an excellent source of 'healthy fat' but is calorific, so eat in moderation. I dip celery and red pepper, sliced as dipping sticks, in guacamole as a treat.

Organic vegetables generally contain more MINERALS such as IRON and ZINC, up to 40% more anti oxidants and have less toxic pesticides on and in them. One way to ensure that you lessen the amount of toxins you ingest is to soak your vegetables in warm water with vinegar and lemon juice, then rinse thoroughly. Your body's liver is constantly sorting through what comes into your body and toxins can accumulate in your system. Consider spending time on a shared allotment. Our soils are depleted so essential minerals may be much lower than they were a generation ago.

The vegetables that are lowest in pesticides are onions, asparagus, sweet peas, eggplant, cabbage, sweet potatoes and mushrooms. The ones that can be high in pesticides are celery, spinach, peppers, white potatoes, lettuce and kale so think about growing your own or buy organic when you can. The more green the vegetable, the more beneficial it will be nutritionally and the ones that top the list are Chinese cabbage, watercress, kale, spinach, the greens from beet, mustard, dandelion and turnip, chicory, romaine and leaf lettuce, chard, endive and chive. Include the brassica group of vegetables

VEGETABLES

every week which are broccoli, Brussels sprouts and cauliflower. (Research this if you have thyroid problems).

Carrots are best eaten cooked, for the body to absorb the nutrients efficiently and I sometimes grate mine, soften in butter then add a small amount of water to cook through. Stir fry, steam or roast your vegetables as microwaves and boiling will reduce the nutrients. If you do steam or boil them, keep the water to make soup.

Some vegetables complement each other in regard to taste and the uptake of vitamins and broccoli and tomatoes are a good team. Tomatoes contain lycopene which can help reduce your chances of developing skin cancer. We badly need some sun on our skin for the beneficial effects of Vitamin D, just don't burn and overdo it.

Fermented vegetables are excellent chelators which mean they remove toxins and heavy metals from your body. I've been buying fermented cabbage and popping a tablespoon into soups at the last minute or having a mouthful as a snack or on a salad. Fermented vegetables contain beneficial microbes for your BOWELS and intestines. This area of your body is hugely important for your overall health, as it's linked to your immune system and produces the neurotransmitter serotonin, which your brain also produces to elevate mood.

JUICING your vegetables will ensure you consume a wide variety in one large glass, to which you can add spiralina or wheatgrass. You'll absorb the vitamins and minerals efficiently so will feel energised and rehydrated. There are lots of juicing books with delicious combinations, so invest in a juicer and chop and change your recipes to get an array of nutrients. Sprouting is another way to eat oxygen rich vegetables and you can either grow your own or buy them at your local health food shop.

It's the synergistic effect of vegetables that will enhance your health. They contain a delicate balance of amino acids which are the protein building blocks of life. Vegetables also contain enzymes that link to HORMONAL health. Polysaccharides, isoflavones and protease inhibitors that exist in vegetables reduce the layers around tumours, to lower the chance of having to deal with cancer. Taking nutritional supplements can be seen as preventative medicine.

If you do have a garden and are growing your own you could try a composter so that you don't waste the peelings and parts of the fruit and vegetables you don't eat. An obscene amount of FOOD is thrown away and wasted daily. The compost you make will be used to feed and nourish the soil in your garden for your next batch of vegetables. Unfortunately, the food we buy from the supermarkets may have been grown in soil that no longer contains optimal levels of MINERALS. By growing your own food or sharing a plot or allotment you lessen the chemical cocktail of pesticides and herbicides which we ingest every week. Those chemicals are detrimental to good health. Invest in a wormery to make compost. Place it out of the sun and mix shredded cardboard in with the vegetable and fruit peelings, green leaves and egg shells. Let the waste go down before you top it up. Avoid putting the outside of onions or citrus fruit peelings in your composter. When it has broken down enough you can sprinkle it over your garden as fertilizer.

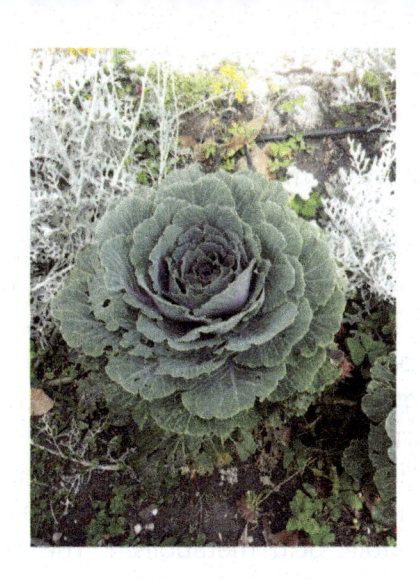

VITAMINS

The soil our fruit and vegetables grow in has been gradually depleted of minerals and some of the food we consume from abroad has been in cold storage for some time before it reaches our tables. Many of my friends devote time and energy to allotments or just a small area in their gardens to grow their own. It makes sense as there are no toxic pesticides involved and you save money. Get some seeds, share a space with friends or get the family working on it as a project.

However diligent you are with food and diet, it's challenging to get the full range of nutrients at levels you need for optimal health. I use Solgar or Higher Nature but there are many companies that supply balanced, synergistic supplements. Ratios and amounts are important so unless you've been to a nutritionist and had tests to show a deficiency, buy a multi vitamin and mineral product as the science has already been done for you. You may need more nutrients during MENOPAUSE or if you've been diagnosed with OSTEOPOROSIS.

Many of us will be deficient at some time in our lives but a multivitamin and mineral supplement is wise. If you are low in Vitamin E, ZINC will also be depleted so you'll be open to infections, as your immune system won't be tiptop and copper levels will increase in your system, causing trouble.

Women in particular need B6 in conjunction with all the B vitamins. If B6 is low it impairs B2 metabolism which then affects folic acid metabolism. This then impairs Vitamin C which means that your absorption of IRON will decrease leading to fatigue. The B Vitamins are essential for energy, as is IRON. Vitamin B3 or nicotinamide helps repair DNA damage caused by UV and sun exposure so may prevent or lessen your chances of developing skin cancer.

Vitamin D regulates calcium and phosphorus absorption, boosts your immune system and builds strong bones, teeth and muscles. If there is a deficiency in Vitamin D it can lead to weakness in muscles and bones, depression, pain sensitivity, gum disease, high blood pressure, fatigue and mood swings as it plays a role in serotonin production. Serotonin is a neurotransmitter in the BRAIN linked to contentment. Ensure you get some sun on your SKIN daily for the benefits of Vitamin D.

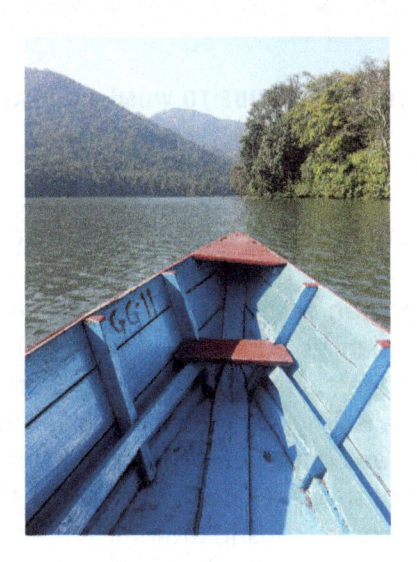

WATER

Water is the most fundamental element in our lives and most of us take it for granted. Millions of people in the world drink dirty, infected water or have to walk miles to a clean source. These people would find it outrageous and incredible that we flush toilets with copious amounts of it. I don't flush my toilet every time, if it's just urine, and I refuse to use bleach in it. Vinegar with lemon and tea tree ESSENTIAL OILS mixed with bicarbonate of soda do a reasonable job of keeping the toilet bowl clean. Access to clean water will become an issue on our planet in the coming years.

We are made up of around seventy percent of water and our bodies and BRAIN need to stay hydrated for optimal health. Limit coffee and sodas, in particular zero cola, as these are detrimental to health, and carry water with you in a glass bottle, not plastic, or a suitable container. If you can't drink enough water in this way, drink herbal teas or weak tea and carry a flask with you.

Healthy, fresh natural food in the form of fruit and vegetables will provide water that is needed to aid the interchange of nutrients in, and waste out, at a cellular level.

If dehydration occurs on a deep level in the cell, we develop imbalances and dis-eases. On our outer layer, this may manifest as dry, itchy SKIN, psoriasis, eczema and brittle nails. There may be hair loss (alopecia), dry, dull hair and eye irritations.

In the digestive area you could suffer from irritable BOWEL syndrome, constipation, ulcers and acid reflux (regurgitation of partially digested food). Water will be taken from your colon and skin to important internal organs. You may also experience SUGAR cravings, blood sugar imbalances and type 2 Diabetes.

Asthma and breathlessness, weight gain, blood pressure and cholesterol issues may manifest. Dehydration is linked to the release of histamine and there may be inflammation and pain in your joints and muscles, as well as headaches and earache.

Eventually, chronic dehydration can affect your mental stability, as insomnia becomes a problem, and you experience mood swings and depression.

Cellular dehydration is not just a lack of water or drinking insufficient quantities of fluid.

Any kind of stress, whether it's physical, mental or emotional will trigger a surge of the HORMONES adrenalin and cortisol. This trigger is known as the "fight or flight" response. When it occurs after a stressful moment, energy is sent to the muscles for an active, physical action in relation to the perceived threat, and your blood becomes thicker and blood pressure is raised. Most of the time these threats do not need to be dealt with by a battle or running away, but the response in the body has created a negative reaction which can leave us feeling constantly anxious and unnerved. Just by thinking about the incident again will trigger the same hormonal reaction in your body, which is why it's important to use MINDFULNESS to ensure you let the experience go. By watching your mind and the train of THOUGHTS, you can decide what you allow yourself to think about. You alone can press the 'stop' button when you realize that you're replaying a scenario over and over in your mind.

Using relaxation in your life will allow you to deactivate from this alerted state. The more stressed you are over a period of time, the more fluid you'll need. Only have one or two coffees early in the day as this heightens the alerted state. Have a few dry nights so that you have red wine and ALCOHOL just a few nights a week. Excessive alcohol consumption leads to further dehydration and has been linked to cancer.

If your brain becomes parched and is dehydrated, your BRAIN chemistry changes your mood. Water is needed to take tryptophan, which is an amino acid, into the brain to produce serotonin. Serotonin is linked to contentment and is a neurotransmitter. It is also produced in a healthy BOWEL.

If you reach a point of chronic dehydration, the outer layer of individual cells, of which there are millions and millions, will develop a 'shell' or coating. This shell is cholesterol and it will prevent the cell from allowing nutrients in, and waste and toxins out.

Dehydration will cause an imbalance in the electrolytes which are needed for electrical impulses between cells and efferent muscle and nerve function. If this imbalance of electrolytes occurs in the blood from a lack of calcium ions, blood ph will drop, and become acidic. For optimal health we need our systems to be predominantly alkaline. We maintain that by eating fresh fruit and VEGETABLES and not eating excessive amounts of protein. An acidic body is one in which disease can manifest as bacteria, fungi and viruses thrive in it.

Make time in your week to practise MEDITATION, YOGA or QIGONG or some form of relaxation that doesn't include junking out on carbohydrates or booze. Have a warm bath occasionally with lavender and chamomile ESSENTIAL OILS. Find a relaxation technique on CD or online and use it nightly. Talk to a friend or counsellor if you feel overwhelmed. Prolonged and constant stress is a potential killer.

Drink filtered water before a meal and during the day and aim, at the very least, for a litre of fluid daily.

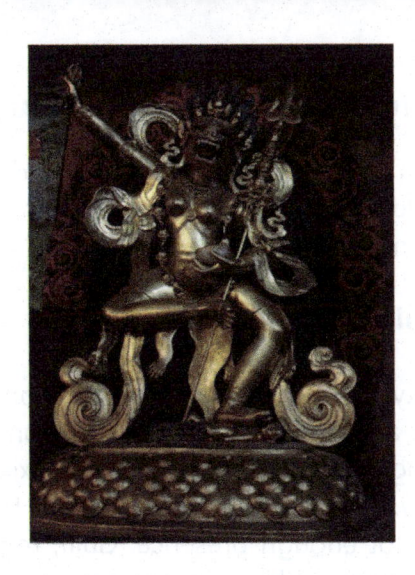

WORDS OF WISDOM

Gandhi's list

Change yourself. Forgive and let go. Take care of this moment. Without action you aren't going anywhere. Everyone is human. See the good in people and help them. Persist. Be congruent, authentic. Be your true self. Grow and evolve.

Paul Ferrini

The simple beauty and majesty of life is to be found in its cyclical rhythms; the rising and setting of the sun, the phases of the moon, the changes in the seasons, the beating of the heart, the rhythmic unfolding of the breath. Repetition provides continuity, familiarity, safety. It is not just the reach of our hands toward the sky, but the rootedness of your feet in the ground that helps you bring heaven to earth. Spirituality is a living with, as well as a living for. It is the poetry of being, the rhythm of life unfolding in each person and each relationship, moment to moment.

Eckhart Toll

All negativity is caused by an accumulation of psychological time and denial of the present. Non acceptance of how things are right now. Unease, anxiety, tension, stress, worry, all forms of fear are caused by too much future and not enough presence. Guilt, regret, resentment, grievances, sadness, bitterness and all forms of non forgiveness are caused by too much past and not enough presence. Your mind is attached to the past and the future. Being present is the key to peace. Use your senses fully. Be where you are. Look around and see the light, shapes, colours, textures. Be aware of the silent presence of each thing. Listen closely. Observe the inner body, your breath, and your emotions. Move deeply into the Now, whatever you're doing.

Buddhist

Try to recognise the precious nature of each day. Like the birds that gather in the treetops at night and scatter in all directions at the coming of dawn, phenomena are impermanent. Nothing is permanent. The sun and the moon rise and then set. The bright clear day is followed by the deep, dark night. From hour to hour, everything changes. Impermanence is a principle of harmony. When we don't struggle against it, we are in harmony with reality. Awareness of impermanence is encouraged so that when it is coupled with our appreciation of the enormous potential of our human existence, it will give us a sense of urgency that I must use every precious moment.

F.Scott Fitzgerald

Start whenever you want. You can change or stay the same. There are no rules to this thing. We can make the best or the worst of it. I hope you make the best of it. I hope you see things that startle you. I hope you feel things you never felt before. I hope you meet people who have a different point of view. I hope you live a life you're proud of, and if you're not, I hope you have the courage to start all over again.

Thich nat han

The present moment is where life can be found, and if you don't arrive there you miss your appointment with life.

Rainer Maria Rilke

My life is not this steeply sloping hour, in which you see me hurrying. Much stands behind me; I stand before it like a tree; I am only one of my many mouths and at that, the one that will be still the soonest. I am the rest between two notes, which are somehow always in discord because death's note wants to climb over, but in the dark interval, reconciled, they stay there trembling. And the song goes on, beautiful.

Buddhist

The near enemy of loving kindness is attachment. At first, attachment may feel like love, but as it grows it becomes more clearly the opposite, characterised by clinging, controlling and fear. The near enemy of compassion is pity, as this also separates us. Pity feels sorry for that person as if he or she were somehow different from us. The near enemy of sympathetic joy (the joy in the happiness of others) is comparison, which looks to see if we have more than, the same as or less than another. The near enemy of equanimity is indifference. True equanimity is balance in the midst of experience, whereas indifference is a withdrawal and not caring, based on fear.

Paul Ferrini

There is always some degree of pain in the release of someone or something that once brought you joy and happiness. You have to be patient and mourn the loss. But when your mourning is over, you will see things differently. Opportunities you never could have dreamed of will come into your life. As the old dies the new is born. The phoenix rises from the ashes of destruction. The fire of change is never easy to weather but if you surrender the conflagration is quickly over. In the enriched soil, the seeds of tomorrow can be sown. When one door is closed, you must wait patiently for another door to open. As long as you forgive yourself and others you won't have to wait long. It isn't helpful to obsess about your mistakes. Guilt doesn't help you act more responsibly to others. Correct your mistakes if you can. Accept things as they are. Make amends to those you have hurt.

Ekhart Toll

Are you worried? Do you have many "what if" thoughts? You are identified with your mind, which is projecting itself into an imaginary future situation and causing fear. There is no way that you can cope with such a situation because it doesn't exist. It's a mental phantom. You can stop this health and life corroding insanity simply by acknowledging the present moment. Become aware of your breathing. Feel your inner body. All that you ever have to deal with, cope with, in real life, as opposed to imaginary mind projections, is this moment. You can always cope with the Now but you can never cope with the future, nor do you have to. The answer, the strength, the right action or resource will be there when you need it, not before, not after.

Sonia Cafe and Neide Inecco

Our greatest release is to free ourselves from attachments of the past and concerns with the future, to be able to live in the present moment. When we do this, we concentrate our energies, and we don't lose vitality by criticizing, comparing and judging. The quality of release frees us from guilt, which is a great waste of energy. Release brings freedom from attachment to possessions or fear of loss.

14th Dalai Lama

We have bigger houses but smaller families; more conveniences but less time; we have more degrees, but less sense; more knowledge but less judgement; more experts, but more problems; more medicines but less healthiness; We've been all the way to the moon and back, but have trouble crossing the street to meet the new neighbour. We build more computers to hold more information to produce more copies than ever, but have less communication; we have become long on quantity, but short on quality. These are the times of fast foods but slow digestion; Tall men but short character; Steep profits but shallow relationships. It's a time when there is much in the window, but nothing in the room.

Rumi

This being human is a guest house, every morning a new arrival. A joy, a meanness, some momentary awareness comes as an unexpected visitor. Welcome and entertain them all! Even if they are a crowd of sorrows who violently sweep your house empty of its furniture, still, treat each guest honourably. He may be clearing you out for some new delight. The dark thought, the shame, the malice, meet them at the door laughing and invite them in. Be grateful for whoever comes, because each has been sent as a guide from beyond.

Lucille Clifton

What will see me through the next twenty years is my knowledge that even in the face of the sweeping away of all that I assumed to be permanent, even when the universe made it quite clear to me that I was mistaken in my certainties, in my definitions, I did not break.

Tao-Te-Ching

Do you have the patience to wait 'til your mud settles and the water is clear? Can you remain unmoving 'til the right action arises by itself? The secret waits for eyes unclouded by longing.

Buddhist

When the mind is full of memories and preoccupied by the future, it misses the freshness of the present moment. In this way we fail to recognise the luminous simplicity of mind that is always present behind the veils of thought. On days when the sky is grey, the sun has not disappeared forever. We can always begin again. Things' falling apart is a kind of testing and also a kind of healing. Learning to live is learning to let go. When there's a disappointment, I don't know if it's the end of the story. It may be just the beginning of a great adventure. Our hearts can grow strong at the broken places.

The Way of Peace Paul Ferrini

The most important door is the one to your heart. If it is open, then the whole universe abides in you. If it is closed, then you stand alone against the world. A heart in resistance gets tired quickly. Life weighs heavily on it. But a heart that is open is filled with energy. It dances and sings. When the door to your heart is open, all the important doors open in the world. You go where you need to go. Nothing interferes with your purpose or your destiny.

XYLITOL

Xylitol is an alternative to SUGAR. It is a low calorie, sugar alcohol sweetener from a plant. As it has 30% fewer calories than sugar and contains fibre, it could be beneficial on a weight loss program. If we want to lose or maintain a certain weight for health reasons we need to cut back on sugar. If you bake regularly, use xylitol or other plant alternatives. The increase in the number of children and teenagers with extreme tooth decay and type 2 diabetes is alarming and linked to our excessive use of sugar.

If you eat a large amount of xylitol over a long period you may experience bloating, flatulence and diarrhea. The other drawback or negative factor regarding xylitol is that it can be "hydrogenated". This means that it goes through a chemical process using hydrogen and a catalyst such as nickel. Hydrogenated foods are linked to degenerative diseases and depression. Use it sparingly.

However, the benefits of using xylitol are probably higher than its drawbacks. It does not have a great effect on blood sugar levels which is a positive factor. It is also thought to combat tooth decay.

Stevia is another alternative to SUGAR and sweeteners. Stevia is taken from the leaves of the plant stevia rebaudiana and is 150 times sweeter than sugar. It comes from South America where it has been used for hundreds of years. It's marketed as Truvia and Rebiana. 4mg/kg of body weight is a safe amount to take daily.

Other alternatives to sugar include the katemfe fruit and thaumatin which is taken from a West African shrub. This is an extremely sweet tasting protein. Luo Han Kuo is from a Chinese fruit and can be used to sweeten food.

Trehalose is a type of natural sugar found in plants and insects. It blocks the process of fructose being stored in the liver as fat and triggers liver cells to get rid of excess fat.

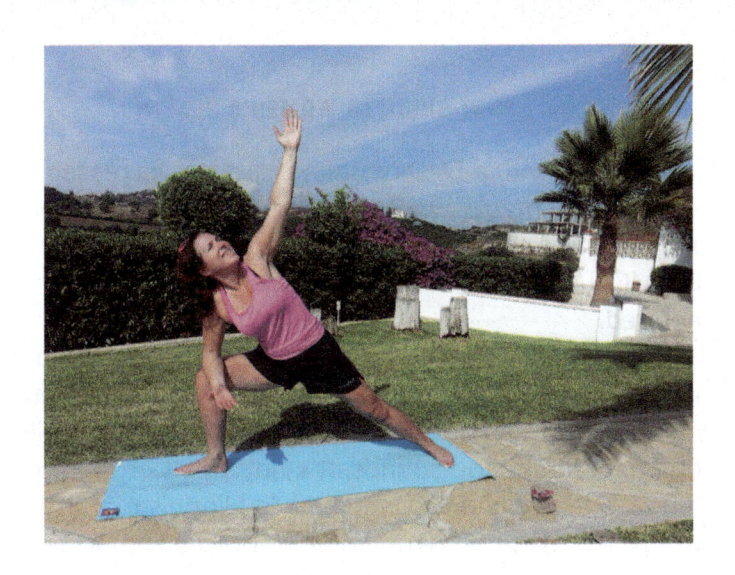

YOGA

The success of yoga does not lie in the ability to perform postures, but in how it positively changes the way we live our life and our relationships. The ultimate goal of yoga is to always observe things accurately and therefore never act in a way that will make us regret our actions later.

T.K.V Desikachar

Master your breath, let the self be in bliss, contemplate on the sublime within you.

T.Krishnamacharya

Yoga is not a stretch. Some people think of it as just a way to lengthen their hamstrings after a long run, and it will do that, but it's much more. Athletes, footballers and celebrities have brought yoga to the forefront of the media in the last couple of decades. The number of people practising it in health clubs and church halls and at home with a DVD or online class has increased. It doesn't really matter why you started. It will benefit your joints, alleviate back pain and balance your endocrine HORMONAL system and leave you feeling calm and centered.

You may have tried it and decided it was too slow and boring for you, or assumed it was just about wrapping your leg around the back of your head while you chanted strange sounds. It's not a cult or religion, although its roots are connected to Hinduism and the ancient language Sanskrit. Yoga embraces and accepts all religions, as we should. There are many paths home.

Yoga has morphed, changed and developed in the few thousand years it's been practised. Recently, companies have mixed it with other disciplines into hybrids. Change is part of life. There are many different schools of yoga and hundreds of thousands of teachers out there with their own style and delivery. Go to different classes and teachers to try them, so that you keep an open mind.

Yoga is a path which can be challenging. Your fascia, joints, muscles and endocrine HORMONAL system will benefit if it's done mindfully without force or expectation. You'll have moments when you realise how it feels to become very still in your mind, as you deeply relax into your body. As you still the mind you start to have an awareness of how it leaps around in the past and future. Practise means to watch the 'thinker' and become an observer. You become aware of thoughts leading into emotions, then reaction. We're human. Let's not pretend, as we practise, that we're perfect and never experience so called negative emotions. The key is to acknowledge and understand. The practise of yoga involves moving beyond chasing pleasure and avoiding pain. To practise yoga is to move towards more of a balanced state and equanimity, and to be more mindful of criticising and judging ourselves and others. It does not involve being sanctimonious when other people 'mess up', or feeling superior, or showing off if you can do the splits while you're upside down in a handstand. It involves Service. Through my life I've struggled with the conundrum of attempting to follow a spiritual path and surrendering, and at the same time, not be walked all over. Any grievances or attempts to hurt you can still be dealt with if you feel they're worth it. Speak your truth clearly and firmly when the time comes. We need to have boundaries in RELATIONSHIPS and guidelines as to what is acceptable to us, and what's not.

In times of grief or strife and agitation yoga can be a still, comforting state in which you are present and accepting. It is a link between the physical body, mind and spirit. If you're ill and exhausted, it is more challenging to stay on a spiritual path, so the postures or asanas enable the body to be as healthy as it can be. What is a spiritual path? It's an inner transformation and connection to something deep within you, and something higher than you, the Divine.

The Yamas and Niyamas are an integral part of yoga practise, along with the postures, pranayama breathing and meditation. Yamas are moral, social and ethical practises. Niyamas are observational, individual disciplines. Yama and Niyama are divided into ten principles or guides. They are a link to mind and behaviour. Yama translates into restraint.

The five guidelines of Yama are; Ahimsa which means non violence, Satya is truth, Asteya is to refrain from stealing and Brahmacharya translates into purity. Aparigraha is non attachment.

The first Yama, ahimsa, non violence, links to your yoga practise where you are gentle with yourself and any limitations, injuries or challenged parts of your body, in your physical practise of yoga.

It also means to live in a way that you don't cause physical or mental, emotional harm to any living being. Thoughts and feelings can be violent if we allow frustration, fear, anger and jealousy to take a hold, and we then react. We can get to the root of why we're feeling that way. We'll still experience these emotions, but awareness will allow us to take a step back and observe if we choose to.

As women we experience fluctuations in HORMONES during puberty, pregnancy, PMS and MENOPAUSE. Maintaining a regular yoga practise with breathing techniques and yoga nidra (deep relaxation) will ensure we take time for ourselves in those challenging weeks or years. I have noticed, to my detriment, that as a yoga teacher, if I neglect my personal practise everything starts to feel off kilter, and events can seem larger and more important than they really are. We can't fully control our physiological systems or surges of hormones or deep fatigue, but we can find ways to restore ourselves. It can be difficult to juggle all the things we do in our week, and to stay steady, and to practise ahimsa when we can. Take a DETOX day when you can.

Be watchful of frustration and resentment building through your life. A DIARY can help with acknowledging events, emotions and triggers. These emotions may be linked to what you see as injustice and unfairness within families, RELATIONSHIPS or at work.

As women, we play different roles or have to perform as an assortment of characters, whilst maintaining our authentic self. We are different things to a myriad of people. We put on our professional heads in our careers and attempt to practise ahimsa within our teams. Then, we mediate with fractious family members, being mindful of not taking sides and trying to be kind in the face of hostility. It can be tough to be thoughtful, compassionate and loving when we're exhausted and have volatile teenagers or overbearing or aging parents. Take time away and be kind to yourself. If you practise ahimsa with yourself, you will be more able to practise it with others.

The next yama is Satya; to be truthful and to avoid lying. One-upmanship can spiral into bragging and exaggerating, so notice what you think and say when you're with a group of people who seem to be competing. It will sometimes be those people who are insecure who feel the need to do this, but avoid judging them. Whenever you can, speak the truth with compassion for the person you're talking to and try to see the good in people generally.

Asteya, or non-stealing is connected to the knowledge that you already have abundance in one form or another. Start to believe that you will always have what you need. Stealing sometimes comes from a feeling of lack and poverty consciousness or desperation. It will also stem from greed and selfishness. Our societies have become more and more obsessed with material bling and shows of wealth. What's inside you is much more important. More and more people are realising this now.

You'll meet people through life who leave you feeling drained and disconcerted. They may insist that they're your friend but talk 'at' you, instead of with you, for hours. They will use you as a sounding board to offload their 'stories' about themselves. This is different to a close friend confiding in you when there is problem. Finding the funny and mutually enjoyable things to do together is what friends are for. People who steal hours of your time and your energy regularly, but do not engage you in mutual conversation, can be very gently released. Be aware of stealing other peoples' energy in this way. When you look around at the world, our problems can seem trivial.

Brahmacharya is the third yama and relates to purity. It also means to be aware of where you direct your energy and the things you choose to focus on. It's not just abstaining from SEX although celibacy is part of its ancient meaning. In our modern daily lives brahmacharya can be applied by staying aware of overt, in your face sexuality. In these times of pornography, advertising, social media and marketing, sex is used to sell and at times, to portray women as sexual objects. If you're a teenager or in your early twenties be mindful of the messages you're sending out regarding what you wear, say and how you act around MEN. Our image and what we wear and how we look can be part of our creativity but may be construed in other ways. We're all naturally sensual and making love in a committed, respectful relationship is a joy. This isn't harking back to Victorian values, just respecting and loving you.

Aparigraha is the next yama and means non attachment. The Sanskrit word apara translates to 'of another', and agraha is to 'crave'. It also means to eliminate excessive accumulation and to avoid hoarding. Fear of loss can relate to a RELATIONSHIP, a feeling of importance or prestige, a job or money. Accept change as and when it happens and move on.

I've been self employed for most of my working life and as a yoga teacher for sixteen years. Some years it's been a challenge to avoid grasping for recognition that I'm competent and for money to pay my bills and to keep my head above water financially.

We seem to have become enamoured with celebrities and their lifestyles, and to feel that we must compete and have more expensive, material items than our neighbours or acquaintances. Practising aparigraha means we watch for feelings of envy and wishes that involve grasping something that belongs to someone else. This also applies to people, chasing someone who isn't available as they are in a RELATIONSHIP with someone else. Before you act always ask yourself how you would feel if someone did the same thing to you.

I have noticed over the years that I'm not envious of diamond rings or expensive cars or designer mansions but of travel experiences, craving to see and experience exotic places around the world. I know I can be content in my own back garden if I choose to be.

It can be challenging to show KINDNESS to everyone in today's world but generosity and understanding are qualities worth cultivating.

The five principles of Niyama are saucha meaning cleanliness, santosha is contentment, tapas relates to austerity and will power and svadhaya is self study. Isvarapranidhana is surrender.

The first niyama is saucha which links into the yama bramacharya. Addiction in society is rife and people need to be shown KINDNESS and understanding if they are dealing with addiction. It may be DRUGS or ALCOHOL or SEX that they're addicted to. People take these stimulants to avoid facing themselves and situations which they find too painful or challenging to address.

We have our bodies on earth for a limited time and need to care for them as we do our minds. That is our responsibility while we're here. A practise that involves MINDFULNESS and MEDITATION, still silence as well as physical movement, will allow us to contemplate purity and to see from a clear mind.

What you think about and what you ingest in the way of food and drink relate to saucha. Being mindful of what you think, feel and say will lead you towards positive thoughts and actions. Don't sweep the negative emotions under the carpet as they are messages that need to be heeded and unravelled. We all want to be happy and to feel peaceful.

I have found the saucha niyama a challenge at times, as have a habit of untidiness and being disorganised. It's still one that I'm working on.

The second Niyama is santosha or contentment. The Sanskrit 'tush' means to be pleased. Contentment links into acceptance of how things are and GRATITUDE for what we have. This means taking steps to realise that outward worldly things, events and people need not dictate whether we are happy or not. In Buddhism, desires lead to suffering as we may not always get what we crave or think we want. The things we chase after are generally temporary and transient but a deep inner peace will sustain you. Our memories and imagination will lead us away from contentment sometimes, as we hanker after something or someone who we felt made us happy.

Tapas is the third Niyama and translates as heat or inner fire, linking to self will and a determined attitude in our regular practise of yoga. In ancient times it related to austerity and now can mean having everything in moderation. Tapas gives us enthusiasm to hone ourselves, then to help others. There's a bright light inside of us, as there is in everyone, but over the years our outer covering can become dusty if not polished and maintained. We are not just our minds or THOUGHTS. Yoga practise allows that light to shine brightly as we use the postures, pranayama (breath control) and MEDITATION and MINDFULNESS.

The fourth Niyama is svadhyaya or self study. Mindfulness is the key to watching the thinker and observing our emotions and reactions, habits and triggers from conditioning. We can start to notice our rigid attitudes or fears and fixed opinions. We start to gently notice when our egos rear up and insist that we are right. It takes a lot of effort to be aware and attentive moment by moment through every day.

Isvarapranidhana translates as surrender to God. Think of yourself as a radiant light inside the vehicle of your body and brain and mind. We have this vehicle for a short time. View a higher divine light or God or whatever you wish to call it, as a constant light in you, around you and connecting all of us and something higher than our earthly existence. The opposite of this is separation and ego and superiority. To surrender takes inner strength, as it means to fully accept life, just as it is, moment by moment. Watch your THOUGHTS constantly as they are seeds that are planted, and become energy that moves into the world. Think of everyone as energy and your thoughts as tangible waves that create your world.

ZINC

Zinc is an essential mineral but many people are deficient in it as bodily stores can be low, so have to be replaced daily with foods such as eggs, sesame and pumpkin seeds, peanuts, brazil nuts, walnuts, popcorn, seafood and sardines or a supplement.

Other nutrients such as calcium, copper and cadmium will be absorbed by the body before it will assimilate zinc. A chemical used in canning will bind to zinc taking it out of the body so limit what you eat from tins.

Zinc forms part of many enzymes and is essential for keeping the immune system healthy as it is needed in the process of assisting the formation of mature, active lymphocytes which are an integral part of the body's immune and defence system. It improves glucose tolerance.

It is also needed for cell growth, testosterone production, sperm formation and sexuality. If you're planning a pregnancy ensure your man is topped up with zinc from the foods above and his multi VITAMIN and MINERAL supplement.

Zinc aids the activity of vitamin D in promoting calcium absorption which is important if you're approaching MENOPAUSE, and need to avoid OSTEOPOROSIS. Zinc also regulates prostaglandins, hormone like substances

ZINC

in the body which, if imbalanced, can exacerbate menstrual cramps.

It's best to take zinc as part of a multi vitamin and mineral supplement. 15 to 50mg a day can be taken. If you only take zinc and nothing else it may disrupt copper metabolism which will disrupt iron metabolism, so a multi supplement will have the required, balanced amounts of each nutrient so they work synergistically.

CONTENTS

A

Airbrushed
Alcohol
Alternatives
Anti Oxidants

B

Bowels
Brain
Breasts

C

Chemicals
Chi
Chocolate
Chylamidia
Coconut Oil and Milk
Contraceptives

D

Debt
Detox
Diary
Drugs

E

Essential Oils
Exercise

F

Fasting
Fertility
Fish
Food

G

Garlic
Genetically Engineered
Goals
Gratitude
Green Tea

A TO Z MINI-GUIDE TO WOMEN'S HEALTH

H

Herbs
Hormones

I

Iron

J

Juicing

K

Kindness

L

Love

M

Meditation
Men
Menopause
Minerals

N

Nuts

O

Omegas
Osteoporosis
Ovaries

P

Products

Q

Qigong

R

Recipes
Relationships

S

Sex
Skin
Sleep
Sugar

T

Thoughts
Toxic

CONTENTS

U

Urinary
Us
Uterus

V

Vagina
Vegetables
Vitamins

W

Water
Words of Wisdom

X

Xylitol

Y

Yoga

Z

Zinc

BIBLIOGRAPHY AND RECOMMENDED READING

Menopause without medicine by Linda Ojeda
The Wisdom of Menopause
by Dr Christiane Northrup
Hot sex by Tracey Cox
The Encyclopaedia of Essential oils by Julia Lawless
The Fragrant Pharmacy by Valerie Ann Worwood
Hormonal Health by Dr Michael Colgan
The New Nutrition by Dr Michael Colgan
Super juice Me by Jason Vale
Anatomy and Physiology by Kathleen J.W Wilson
Insight Yoga by Sarah Powers
The Yoga book by Stephen Sturgess
The complete illustrated book of yoga
by Swami Vishnu-devander
The Bhagavad Gita by Ecknath Easwaren
The Way of Qigong by Kenneth S. Cohen
Was it something you ate?
By John Emsley and Peter Fell
The 30 Day Fat Burner Diet by Patrick Holford
The Sirtfood diet recipe book
by Aidan Goggins and Glen Matten.
The Power of Now by Eckhart Tolle
Queen bees and Wannabees by Rosalind Wiseman
The 5:2 Diet Book by Kate Harrison

A TO Z MINI-GUIDE TO WOMEN'S HEALTH

WEBSITES

www.drmercola.com
www.wddty.com
webmd.com
www.lauralefkowitzmd.com

ACKNOWLEDGEMENTS

Thank you to my parents Julie and Dave Mckay for their proofreading and technical help. Gratitude and thanks to Sean Mullin (Perception websites) for always being there to advise and support me on my website and for designing my book cover. Elly Hush gave me advice and informed me of the procedures and details of university finances, so thank you for your help.